Mechanical Ocular Trauma

Hua Yan
Editor

Mechanical Ocular Trauma

Current Consensus and Controversy

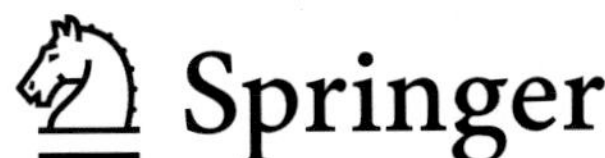

Editor
Hua Yan
Department of Ophthalmology
Tianjin Medical University General Hospital
Tianjin, China

ISBN 978-981-10-9542-9 ISBN 978-981-10-2150-3 (eBook)
DOI 10.1007/978-981-10-2150-3

Printed on acid-free paper

This Springer imprint is published by Springer Nature
The registered company is Springer Science+Business Media Singapore Pte Ltd.
The registered company address is 152 Beach Road, #22-06/08 Gateway East, Singapore 189721, Singapore

Preface

Ocular trauma is the leading cause of blindness in young people. The treatment is complex and often requires combined surgeries or multiple procedures. In the era of precision medicine, precise medical diagnosis and personalized treatment are required to every single patient which put forward higher requirements to ophthalmologists. Accurate timing of surgery and the rational use of drugs and surgical techniques are the crux to save visual function in patients with ocular trauma.

With the development of science and medical technology, many previously controversial issues in the field of ocular trauma have reached consensuses in a certain degree. However, some of the issues still have strong arguments and remain controversial. It is such dispute we urge the deepening understanding of the disease. It is also such dispute we keep improving our service to the patients with ocular trauma, providing better health care. Hence, the focus of this book is on hot topics in the field of ocular trauma, from a new perspective. This book presents the state-of-the-art consensuses and controversies. It is expected that this book can help ophthalmologists to fully understand the latest progress in this field and to promote the development of the ocular trauma field through discussion of the controversial issues.

The authors of this book are top-rated doctors and professors from around the world, including:

- Hua Yan, MD, PhD*; Jiaxing Wang, MD; Caiyun You, MD, PhD; Xiangda Meng, MD, PhD; Yuanyuan Liu, MD; Song Chen, MD (Chap. 1 and 4)
- Richard K. Lee, MD, PhD*; Mohamed S. Sayed, MD (Chap. 2)
- William E. Smiddy, MD, PhD* (Chap. 3)
- Sengul Ozdek, MD*; M. Cuneyt Ozmen, MD, FICO (Chap. 5)
- Gokhan Gurelik, MD*; Sabahattin Sul, MD (Chap. 6)
- Haoyu Chen, MD, PhD*; Honghe Xia; Danny Siu-Chun Ng (Chap. 7)
  *corresponding author

They are not only the top experts in their fields, but also well-experienced surgeons. Their practicing experience covers Asia, the United States, and European countries whose standpoints are expected to be widely recognized by the international ophthalmology society. However, there may be doctors holding different points of view to this book. We highly value such opinions and sincerely hope to hear such feedbacks. This will be the greatest encouragement and help to the authors of the book, as well as the readers, and also the most valuable asset to the academic world.

This book intends to highlight the awareness and thinking on hot topics through multiple clinical cases with delicate pictures, which are considered to be the most welcomed form to doctor readers. The authors sincerely encourage the readers to offer their valuable comments and suggestions.

Finally, I expect this book can help ophthalmologists to provide better health care and services to patients with ocular trauma. There will be nothing more delightful than seeing the patients regain their eyesight and re-enjoy the beautiful world.

Tianjin, China Hua Yan

Acknowledgment

We hereby acknowledge the following ophthalmologists for providing precious and delicate photos to this book: Jinhong Cai, MD; Haibo Li, MD; Dan Hu, MD; and Zhiliang Wang MD. I also would like to thank Jiuying Zhang for drawing all the operation schematic diagrams and Jiaxing Wang, MD, for his dedication in editing and organizing the photos.

Contents

1 Introduction

Hua Yan, Yuanyuan Liu, and Song Chen

1.1 Introduction

Ocular trauma remains a leading cause of monocular visual loss and blindness and often affects young individuals, especially the most common cause in the pediatric groups. The vision loss caused by ocular trauma not only affects a person's quality of life but also imposes enormous socioeconomic and psychological impacts on patients and their families. By now, great advances have been attained on the management of ocular injuries under the guidelines of the retrospective reviews based on the uniform categories and outcome assessment system for the ocular trauma. In order to make a better analysis of ocular trauma including researches or clinical researches, of great importance seems to make a consensus on the terminology classification, evaluation, and therapeutic interventions for the ocular trauma, which is illustrated in this chapter.

H. Yan, MD, PhD (✉) • Y. Liu, MD • S. Chen, MD
Department of Ophthalmology, Tianjin Medical University General Hospital, Tianjin, China
e-mail: phuayan2000@163.com

1.2 Terminology and Classification of Mechanical Ocular Trauma [BETT Terminology, OTCS (Ocular Trauma Classification System)]

Trauma can cause an extensive damage to the orbit, eyeballs, adnexa, and optic nerve to some extent, which ranges from the superficial lesions to vision loss. Our comprehension of ocular trauma has increased tremendously in the past 100 years, leading to numerous advances in the management of such disease. It is essential for the ophthalmologists and non-ophthalmologists to use a standardized classification system of terminology and assessment when they explain eye condition to the patients, communicate clinical findings with colleague, and do related researches.

1.3 Birmingham Eye Trauma Terminology (BETT) [1]

BETT has been endorsed by a large number of organizations, including the American Academy of Ophthalmology, International Society of Ocular Trauma, US Eye Injury Registry and its 25 international affiliates, Retina Society,

H. Yan (ed.), *Mechanical Ocular Trauma*, DOI 10.1007/978-981-10-2150-3_1

Table 1.1 Terms and definitions in BETT

Term	Definition and comment
Closed globe injury	There is no full-thickness wound on the eyeball (sclera and cornea)
Lamellar laceration	Partial-thickness wound of the eyeball. The wound is just "into" rather than "through"
Contusion	No full-thickness wound of the eyeball. The ocular contusions result from blunt energy delivered directly by some objects (like a fist, balls, doors, stone, or falling on the floor) or shock wave from them. The blunt trauma induces deformation of the globe, which causes the severe traction to the intraocular structures and rupture of tissues, bleeding (e.g., hyphema), and dislocation of normal structures (e.g., angle recession)
Open globe injury	There is at least one wound of full thickness on the eyeball (sclera and cornea)
Rupture	Full-thickness wound of the eyeball is due to blunt energy caused by some blunt object. The blunt force exerts significant impact on the globe resulting in the temporary increase of intraocular pressure, which causes the global rupture at its weakest points (e.g., impact site or limbus). The mechanism of the rupture is actually caused by an inside-out force
Laceration	Full-thickness wound occurs at the impact site caused by a sharp agent, in which an outside-in mechanism is involved
Penetrating injury	Injury of the eyeball has an entrance, but no exit, accompanied by the foreign body retained in the globe. If there are over one wound appeared, each of them must be induced by different objects
IOFB	Injury with one or more than one foreign agent present in the globe, which technically occurs along with the penetrating injury, not separately
Perforating injury	Injury of the eyeball has both entrance and exit caused by the same object

Reprinted with permission from Kuhn [2]

Vitreous Society, and World Eye Injury Registry. The key point of this system is to make distinct definitions referring to the integral globe instead of the specific tissue, for the specified tissue stands for the location rather than a modifier of the term. However, there are some injuries that occur in complicated mechanisms. For instance, if the patient falls down and is hurt by some sharp stuff, the wound should be a laceration which is a common type of penetrating injury, but a concomitant rupture (i.e., loss of eye tissue) with varying degrees of contusion to the retina might be considered in the injury as well. In such example, ocular rupture, as the most serious injury type, is the most appropriate description for the outcomes and implications of the case and also gives a distinct guide for the therapy and prognosis (Table 1.1, Figs. 1.1 and 1.2).

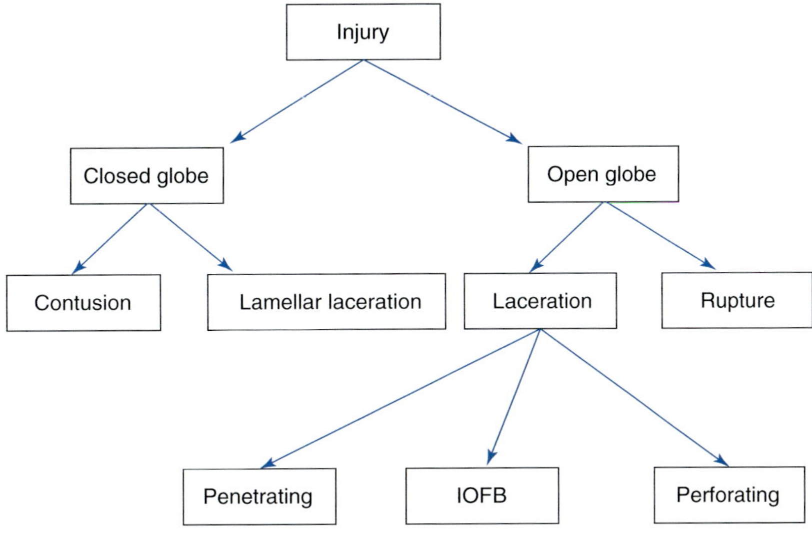

Fig. 1.1 BETT. The bold boxes show the diagnoses that are used in clinical practice (Reprinted with permission from Kuhn [2])

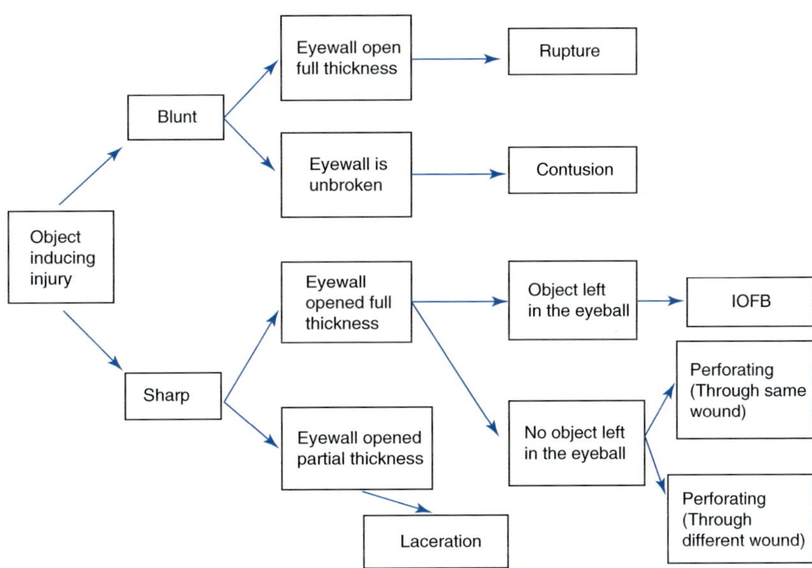

Fig. 1.2 Classification of mechanical eye injuries in BETT used for clinical guidance (Reprinted with permission from Kuhn [2])

Using BETT in ocular traumatology is a mandatory standard to keep unambiguity among the healthcare professionals, without consideration of confusions caused by the communications.

1.4 Classification of Ocular Trauma

In ocular trauma classification developed by the Ocular Trauma Classification Group, mechanical trauma to the eyes is divided into open and closed globe injuries (Table 1.2) [3]. Four separate elements are under consideration: type, grade, presence/absence of a relative afferent pupillary defect (RAPD), and extent of the injury. This classification system will categorize ocular injuries as soon as the ophthalmologists start the initial examination. It is designed to promote the use of standard terminology and assessment, with applications to clinical management and research studies regarding eye injuries [4, 5].

1.5 Ocular Trauma Score (OTS)

Based on BETT, Kuhn and his colleagues analyzed more than 2500 eye injuries from the US and Hungarian Eye Injury Registries and established a model for the evaluation of prognosis in the clinic, named the Ocular Trauma Score (OTS) [6], which predicts the visual outcome of the patients who suffered traumatic ocular injuries. There are six variables involved in the parameters of the OTS, i.e., initial visual acuity, globe rupture, endophthalmitis, perforating injury, retinal detachment, and RAPD, which are assigned to certain numerical values in OTS to make it possible to attain a range of visual acuities after ocular trauma. Although limited variables and basic mathematics are used in OTS, it provides the ophthalmologists an approximately 77 % chance to make a prediction about the eventual functional outcome within ± one visual category timely when the patients arrive the emergency room. The early prognostic information we get from OTS allows an appropriate evaluation of patients and contributes to correct therapeutic strategies made (Table 1.3).

Table 1.2 Ocular trauma classification system (OTCS)

	Open globe injury classification	Close globe injury classification
Type	Rupture Penetrating Intraocular foreign body Perforating Mixed	Contusion Lamellar laceration Superficial foreign body Mixed
Visual acuity[a]	≥20/40 20/50–20/100 19/100–5/200 4/200 to light perception No light perception	≥20/40 20/50–20/100 19/100–5/200 4/200 to light perception No light perception
Pupil condition	RAPD(+) RAPD(−)	RAPD(+) RAPD(−)
Zone (Fig. 1.3)	I: Wounds occur limited to the cornea (corneoscleral limbus included) II: Wounds occur 5 mm posterior to the corneoscleral limbus III: Wounds occur posterior to the anterior 5 mm of the sclera	I: Injuries involve the external structures (confined to the bulbar conjunctiva, sclera, and cornea) II: Injuries involve the internal structures in anterior segment (from the cornea to the posterior lens capsule with the pars plicata included) III: Injuries involve the posterior segment structures posterior to the posterior lens capsule (e.g., retina, macular)

[a]Vision should be measured at a distance of 20 ft using Snellen chart or moved to 3 ft when the symbols can't be discerned, with related lens correction (e.g., myopia, astigmatism) and pinhole when pupil dilated. Make sure the fellow eye well is covered thoroughly during the vision test

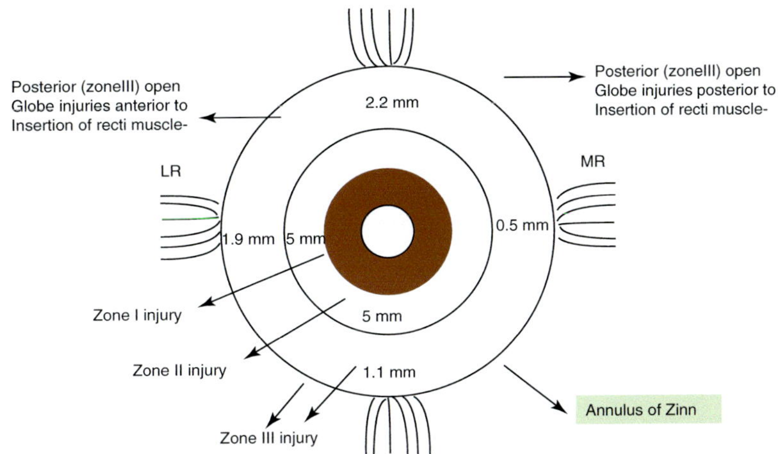

Fig. 1.3 Zones of injuries in open-global and close-global traumas

Table 1.3 Ocular Trauma Score (OTS)

Step 1	Variables used	Raw points				
A	Initial vision					
	NLP	60				
	LP/HM	70				
	1/200–19/200	80				
	20/200–20/50	90				
	≥20/40	100				
B	Perforating injury	−14				
C	Retinal detachment	−11				
D	APD	−10				
E	Rupture	−23				
F	Endophthalmitis	−17				
Step 2. Calculation on the sum of the raw points: A + B + C + D + E + F						
Step 3. Convert the raw points into the OTS and calculate the probability of the ultimate visual categories						
Sum of the raw points	OTS	NLP %	LP/HM %	1/200–19/200 %	20/200–20/50 %	≥20/40 %
0–44	1	74	15	7	3	1
45–65	2	27	26	18	15	15
66–80	3	2	11	15	31	41
81–91	4	1	2	3	22	73
92–100	5	0	1	1	5	94

References

1. Kuhn F, Morris R, Witherspoon CD, Heimann K, Jeffers JB, Treister G. A standardized classification of ocular trauma. Ophthalmology. 1996;103(2):240–3.
2. Kuhn F. Ocular traumatology. Springer; Springer-Verlag Berlin Heidelberg;2008.
3. Bullock JD, Warwar RE. A system for classifying mechanical injuries of the eye (globe). Am J Ophthalmol. 1998;125(4):565–6.
4. De Juan Jr E, Sternberg Jr P, Michels RG. Penetrating ocular injuries: types of injuries and visual results. Ophthalmology. 1983;90(11):1318–22.
5. Groessl S, Nanda SK, Mieler WF. Assault-related penetrating ocular injury. Am J Ophthalmol. 1993;116(1):26–33.
6. Kuhn F, Maisiak R, Mann L, Mester V, Morris R, Witherspoon CD. The ocular trauma score (OTS). Ophthalmol Clin North Am. 2002;15(2):163–5.

2 Anterior Segment Trauma

Richard K. Lee and Mohamed S. Sayed

2.1 Introduction

Mechanical ocular trauma involving the anterior segment may result in damage to the conjunctiva, cornea, limbus, anterior chamber angle, iris, lens, and ciliary body. The mechanism of trauma (closed or open, blunt, penetrating, or perforating), force and extent of trauma, and whether a foreign body is involved determine the pathophysiologic consequence of injury to the various anterior segment structures. The treatment modalities employed and the final visual outcome are also dependent upon these trauma variables. Thorough history taking and careful clinical examination are crucial in the proper assessment and management of anterior segment trauma.

Ocular trauma may be isolated or occur in the context of polytrauma. Systemic evaluation of the patient with attention to vital signs, mental status, and serious or life-threatening non-ocular trauma is indispensable before proceeding with ocular evaluation. This triaging process will direct the decision whether the patient should be evaluated in a general trauma center or in a specialized eye emergency room.

R.K. Lee, MD, PhD (✉) • M.S. Sayed, MD
Department of Ophthalmology, Bascom Palmer Eye Institute, University of Miami, Miami, FL, USA
e-mail: rlee@med.miami.edu

2.2 History

The patient's past medical and surgical history as well as medication history, allergies, past ophthalmic history (including pre-trauma visual acuity (VA)), previous eye surgeries, symptoms of bleeding diathesis, blood dyscrasia or coagulopathy (bleeding gums on tooth brushing, epistaxis, bloody stools), history of complications related to anesthesia, and the time when the patient last ate or drank should be documented.

An updated tetanus immunization status should be determined by the clinician. Intramuscular administration of tetanus immunoglobulin is considered in cases of high-risk open globe injury as confirmed by ocular examination in patients who have not been immunized against tetanus or in patients in whom tetanus immunization status cannot be determined. Intramuscular or subcutaneous administration of tetanus toxoid may be considered in patients who had not received a booster dose within the last 10 years. However, routine tetanus prophylaxis is not recommended in patients with non-open globe injuries [1].

The mechanism of injury and circumstances of the incident as reported by the patient or witnesses should be documented. Blunt trauma usually results in different pathophysiologic processes compared with trauma by sharp objects, and the differentiation between the two based on history taking can guide clinical examination and management. For instance,

H. Yan (ed.), *Mechanical Ocular Trauma*, DOI 10.1007/978-981-10-2150-3_2

blunt trauma warrants careful gonioscopy to detect subtle cases of angle recession and ciliary body detachment secondary to shear forces more prominent in blunt compared to sharp ocular trauma. Additionally, blunt trauma may result in an occult open globe injury (ruptured globe) where the wound site may be hidden by bleeding underneath an intact bulbar conjunctiva or is situated posterior to the insertion of the extraocular muscles (EOMs) which makes direct examination difficult. On the contrary, the laceration site is usually more visible on slit lamp examination when ocular trauma is inflicted by a sharp object resulting in an open globe injury.

The mechanism of injury and whether protective eyewear was worn at the time of injury may also direct the clinician's attention to the possible presence of a foreign body (FB) embedded onto the ocular surface or into intraocular structures that can be overlooked on slit lamp examination, such as in cases of hammering on a nail. Furthermore, the physical setting of trauma may influence the prognosis and final visual outcome, since open globe injuries in a rural setting have a much higher rate of intraocular infection and endophthalmitis [2]. Determining the exact time of injury and the time span between trauma and presentation is also imperative in planning the intervention, particularly in open globe injuries, since a more conservative approach may be employed in certain cases (such as small self-sealing corneal wounds) in which the eye has been quiescently stable for a relatively long period. Moreover, complications such as angle recession glaucoma can often develop years following ocular contusion [3], and regular follow-up visits in patients with suspected injury to the anterior chamber angle should be scheduled for evaluation and early detection of glaucoma. Proper documentation of the mechanism of injury and the circumstances surrounding the incident may also be of medicolegal importance, especially when the clinician's expert opinion is sought or in cases where issues of liability or compensation become relevant.

2.3 Clinical Examination

Upon initial presentation, prompt placement of a protective eye shield and avoidance of eye patching when ocular examination is not being carried out are strongly recommended when open globe injury is suspected.

Visual acuity of both eyes should be assessed early in the evaluation process of the mechanical ocular trauma patient. Visual field screening with the confrontation test is also important and may be predictive of the nature and location of injury. Inspection of the external appearance of the face and periocular tissues may provide important clues to the extent of the injury. For example, gross enophthalmos and periorbital ecchymosis may denote orbital wall fracture, and lacerations involving the eyelid margin are often associated with corneoscleral lacerations and open globe injuries.

Gross inspection without magnification assisted by a flashlight may also reveal the presence of a visible foreign body embedded onto the ocular surface or protruding from the eye, prolapse of uveal tissue and/or other intraocular contents, or pupillary deformity. These observations often suggest, or confirm, the presence of an open globe injury and may necessitate the placement of a protective shield before proceeding with history taking and further evaluation. The presence of large periorbital ecchymosis or eyelid edema may preclude adequate ocular examination, and obtaining imaging studies directly in cases in which open globe injuries cannot be ruled out is safer than exerting undue pressure on the globe to open the eyelids, with possible extrusion of intraocular contents, especially while placing a lid speculum or a Desmarres lid retractor. Assessment of ocular motility, while useful in cases of orbital wall fractures, may also pose a strain on an open globe and is better avoided when suspicion of such injuries is high.

Palpation of the periorbital structures may reveal subcutaneous crepitus, orbital rim deformity, or hypoesthesia/altered sensation in the distribution of the infraorbital nerve, suggesting an associated orbital wall fracture.

2.4 Hot Topics in Mechanical Ocular Trauma Involving the Anterior Segment

2.4.1 Traumatic Iris Injury

The nature of iris involvement in mechanical ocular trauma depends on whether trauma is blunt (open or closed globe) or penetrating. Blunt, closed globe injuries can result in traumatic mydriasis from iris sphincter rupture, while open globe injuries (whether due to blunt or penetrating trauma) can result in iris laceration; iris prolapse through corneal, limbal, scleral, or corneoscleral wounds; and traumatic aniridia. Iridodialysis can also occur secondary to either open globe or closed globe injuries.

2.4.2 Traumatic Mydriasis (Iris Sphincter Rupture)

Traumatic sphincter rupture can be induced by blunt trauma to the eye and can be either temporary or permanent. When persistent, associated mydriasis may cause blurring of vision, halos, glare, night vision symptoms, and poor cosmetic appearance. Pupillary reaction may be sluggish or absent, and radial tears involving the pupillary margin may be observed on slit lamp examination and may be accompanied by traumatic hyphema. Secondary scarring may further limit pupil motility. Differentiating traumatic iris sphincter rupture from preexisting mydriasis secondary to other causes (e.g., pharmacologic dilation, congenital aniridia, iridocorneal endothelial (ICE) syndromes, oculomotor palsy, or anterior proliferative vitreoretinopathy (PVR) with vitreous or fibrovascular strands anchored to the pupillary margin) is important (Fig. 2.1).

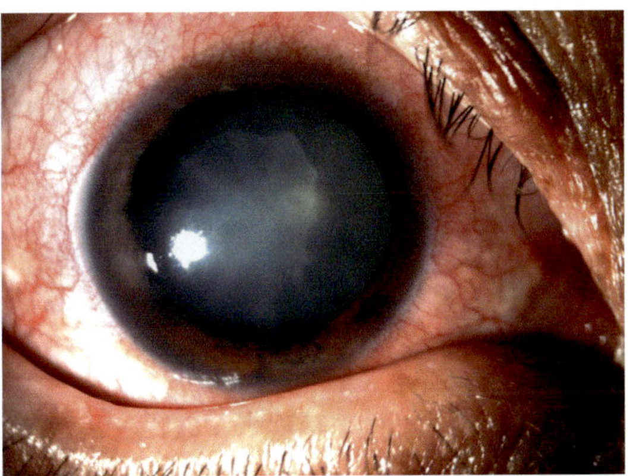

Fig. 2.1 Traumatic mydriasis

No treatment for traumatic mydriasis is necessary in the absence of visually disturbing or cosmetic symptoms. In symptomatic patients, miotic agents such as 1–2 % pilocarpine eye drops four times daily may be attempted. However, pilocarpine is often ineffective and may induce eye pain and/or headache, myopic shift, miosis, reduction of accommodative amplitude, or retinal detachment in predisposed eyes. The use of competitive α-adrenergic antagonists may be better tolerated, with less effect on accommodation and a less frequent dosing schedule [4].

Failure of pharmacologic treatment in symptomatic patients may warrant the use of opaque, iris-print contact lenses to ease the burden of visual symptoms and provide an acceptable cosmetic appearance. However, in case of contact lens intolerance or unsuitability or in cases in which surgical intervention is planned for coexisting traumatic ocular injuries (e.g., traumatic cataract and/or lens subluxation/dislocation), surgical correction of traumatic mydriasis could be considered. Surgical iridoplasty can be achieved by radially cutting the iris extending from the iris periphery to the pupillary margin at the point of presumed sphincter rupture using a pair of iris scissors, followed by bringing the two ends of the cut pupillary border apposed with a permanent 9–0 or 10–0 polypropylene suture using the Siepser slipknot technique (described below in the Sect. 2.4.3, Fig. 2.2). The procedure is repeated distally along the length of the radial iris cut. A running suture acting as an encircling band may also be weaved through the iris margin in a purse string fashion, tied, and tightened as necessary forming a type of pupillary cerclage [5].

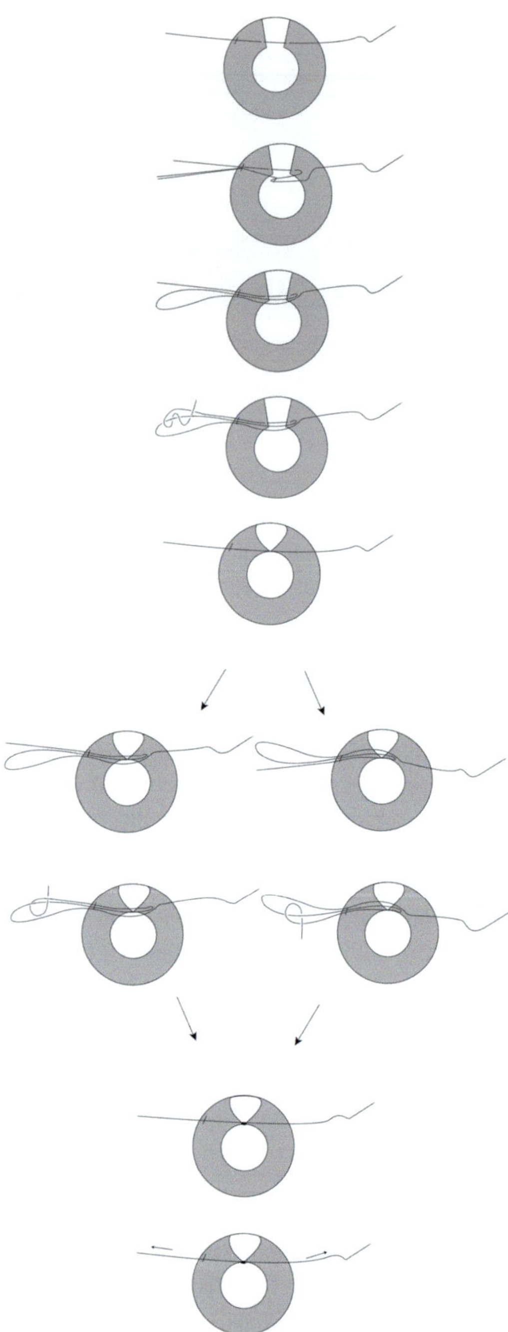

Fig. 2.2 Seipser slipknot technique. Two opposing side ports are made and a 10-0 suture with a CIF-4 needle passed from the first paracentesis through the 2 edges of the iris laceration and externalized out of the second side port incision. The needle is cut and a large loop of suture is pulled out of the entry side port incision intraocularly then out of the second side port incision. A double throw slipknot is made by tying the loop around the free suture end and the knot is slid into the anterior chamber by pulling the 2 suture ends firmly. The process is repeated to form a square knot. The suture ends are trimmed using intraocular scissors

2.4.3 Traumatic Iris Lacerations

Traumatic iris lacerations (Fig. 2.3) can result secondary to penetrating ocular trauma or be iatrogenic (e.g., during cataract surgery where a tuft of iris tissue is caught in the phacoemulsification tip, particularly in cases of floppy iris syndrome). Iris lacerations can result in intraocular bleeding, poor pupillary reaction, mydriasis, poor cosmesis with an eccentric pupil, and visual symptoms similar to those associated with traumatic sphincter rupture and possible associated mydriasis. Large iris lacerations can result in monocular diplopia if traumatic polycoria is present. Iris lacerations may also be associated with other iris deformities (e.g., iridodialysis) and traumatic ocular injuries.

Management of traumatic iris lacerations depends on the extent of injury and whether it is symptomatic. Surgical repair of iris lacerations can be achieved by suturing the two cut ends with a Siepser slipknot (Fig. 2.2) using a permanent 9–0 or 10–0 polypropylene suture on a long needle (e.g., CIF-4 needle, Ethicon) [6]. Two side ports are made at either ends of a projected imaginary line perpendicular to the iris laceration along the suture tract. The needle is then introduced into the anterior chamber through a side port, while a 25-gauge cannula is introduced through the opposite side port to provide countertraction necessary for passing the needle into the iris tissue and for docking the needle tip. The needle is then externalized through the second side port, and the needle is cut leaving long suture

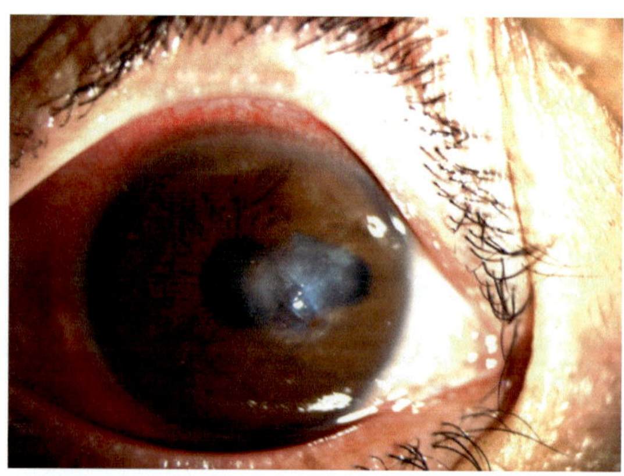

Fig. 2.3 Traumatic iris laceration

ends on both sides. A large loop of suture is then pulled inside the eye and pulled out of the entry side port using a hook (i.e., Bonds or Sinskey). A double throw slipknot is formed by tying the externalized loop around the free suture end and then pulling both suture ends gently and securely to form a slipknot inside the anterior chamber. The process is then repeated to form a square knot. The suture ends are then trimmed short using a pair of intraocular microscissors. If the laceration is large and requires multiple knots along its length, the more proximal ends near the pupillary border should be apposed first and the procedure then repeated distally as required along the laceration length.

2.4.4 Iris Prolapse

Iris prolapse occurs secondary to an open globe injury (due to a blunt force or a penetrating trauma) (Fig. 2.4). The iris tissue may prolapse through corneal, limbal, scleral, or corneoscleral lacerations and can be associated with traumatic iris laceration, iridodialysis, or other ocular injuries. Prompt, timely management of iris prolapse is crucial to store the anatomic integrity of the eye. Delayed management may result in iridocorneal adhesions with ischemia and necrosis of the iris tissue, introduction of microorganisms with the secondary occurrence of endophthalmitis, surface epithelialization and epithelial downgrowth, and peripheral anterior synechia (PAS) formation with secondary angle-closure glaucoma. Surgical management is indicated in all cases in which adequate conjunctival and scleral coverage is present. Surgical management of cases in which iris tissue prolapses through a scleral laceration but is covered by the intact conjunctiva should still be considered when the scleral wound is relatively large because of future extension of the scleral wound and progressive uveal prolapse with blunt force, which may also lead to progressive PAS formation and secondary glaucoma.

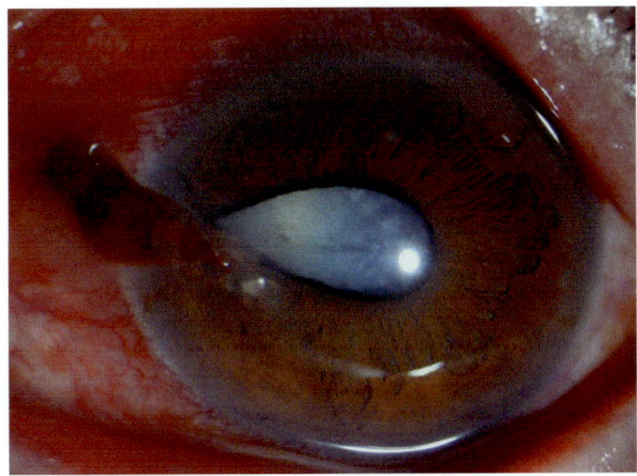

Fig. 2.4 Iris prolapse

Topical and systemic antibiotics should be considered on presentation depending on the extent, length of time, and other ocular risk factors for infection, including consideration of system risk factors such as a compromised immune system. Intracameral antibiotics may be administered intraoperatively to minimize the risk of endophthalmitis. The surgical technique employed depends on the location of the incarcerated iris tissue, anterior chamber depth, duration of prolapse, and viability of the prolapsed iris tissue. Cases in which the location of iris prolapse is peripheral and the anterior chamber is relatively formed can be managed with intracameral administration of mitotic agents (e.g., acetylcholine) through a side port incision with gentle stroking of the prolapsed iris tissue into the eye. Conversely, intracameral injection of mydriatic agents (e.g., epinephrine) may help relieve a small, central iris prolapse. Such simple maneuvers may reposition the prolapsed iris in situ without unnecessary intraocular manipulation.

The intracameral injection of viscoelastic agents through a paracentesis incision to mechanically dislodge and reposit the prolapsed iris tissue into the anterior chamber with or without the aid of a cyclodialysis spatula can be attempted when pharmacologic agents alone fail. Care should be exercised to not exert undue force on the iris root which can result in iatrogenic iridodialysis.

When iris prolapse is relatively long-standing (e.g., >36–48 h), the prolapsed iris tissue should be carefully examined for signs of necrosis or epithelialization. Any unviable iris tissue should be excised without pulling excessively on viable iris. Closure of the resultant iris defect is usually done to avoid monocular diplopia and can be performed utilizing the technique used for traumatic iris lacerations. Globe integrity is then restored by suturing the corneal, limbal, scleral, or corneoscleral wound closed.

2.4.5 Traumatic Iridodialysis

Iridodialysis represents detachment of the iris root from its ciliary insertion (Fig. 2.5). Iridodialysis can result from blunt or penetrating ocular trauma or be inflicted iatrogenically during intraocular surgery. Small iridodialyses or those adequately covered by the upper eyelid are usually asymptomatic. Symptoms of larger iridodialyses include monocular diplopia, glare, and cosmetic disfigurement. Iridodialysis can coexist with other traumatic ocular injuries, including lens subluxation/dislocation and/or vitreous prolapse.

When small, iridodialysis can be managed with frequent instillation of mydriatic eye drops (e.g., atropine) and/or dark sunglasses to reduce light-induced miosis. These measures may result in spontaneous reattachment [7]. Several surgical techniques have been described to correct large iridodialyses. Any vitreous strands prolapsing through the iridodialysis defect should be cut using anterior vitrectomy through a limbal approach prior to suture placement. The most widely used techniques utilize the McCannel technique (Fig. 2.6) [8, 9]. In one modification of the technique, a conjunctival peritomy is made, followed by placing several evenly spaced, full-thickness 1-mm-wide scleral incisions using a microvitreoretinal (MVR) blade, 1 mm behind the limbus along the circumference of

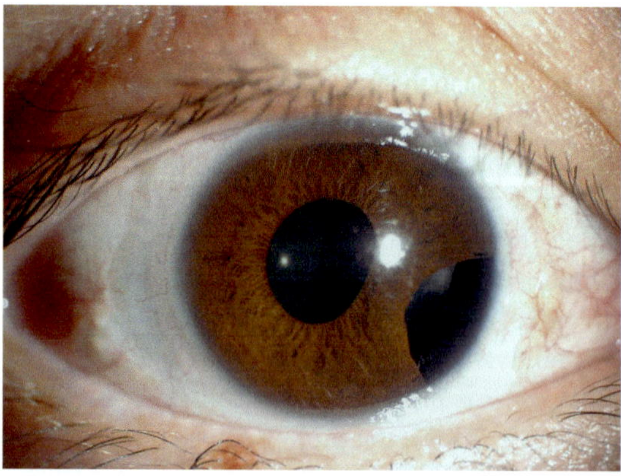

Fig. 2.5 Iridodialysis

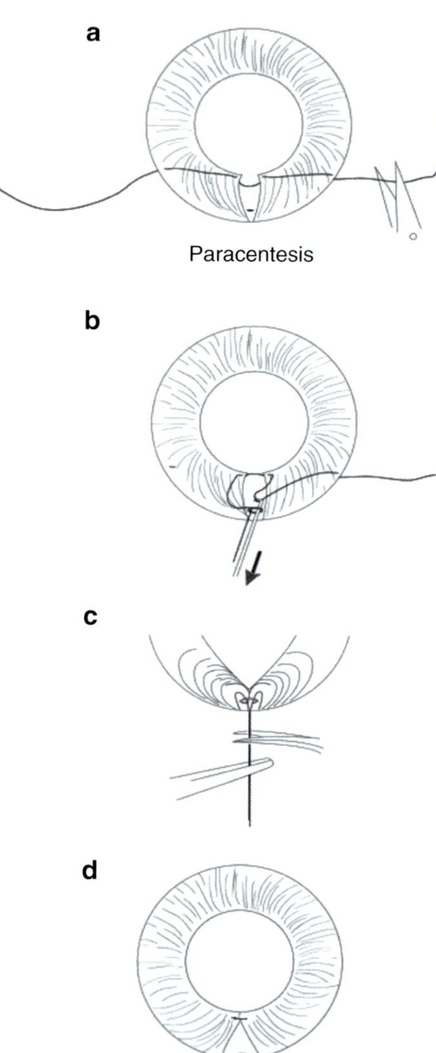

Fig. 2.6 McCannel iris suture technique. (**a**). Creation of 2 opposing side ports using MVR blade, passage of a single-armed 10-0 suture through the 2 edges of iris, and cutting off needle. (**b**). Exteriorization of the 2 suture ends (**c**). Suture ends tied extraocularly and cut flush. (**d**). Sutured iris ends reposited intraocularly

the iridodialysis. Viscoelastic agents are injected through a corneal side port incision in order to push the peripheral edge of the iris distally. Iris hooks may be used if the peripheral iris edge has retracted too far centrally. A long needle with a permanent 10–0 polypropylene suture is then passed through one a previously made sclerotomy to catch the peripheral iris edge and is then externalized through a limbal side port incision or another sclerotomy. The 2 suture ends are externalized using a hook (Bonds or a Sinskey) through a third, central side port and tied together extraocularly, cut flush, and then reposited intraocularly. The procedure can be repeated as necessary depending on the size of iridodialysis. All sclerotomies are then sutured closed.

Another popular technique also involves placing several (at least 2) evenly spaced sclerotomies with the MVR blade 1-mm behind the limbus. A long single-armed needle with a permanent 10–0 polypropylene suture is then passed through a limbal incision across the pupil from the site of iridodialysis to catch the peripheral edge of the iris with the needle tip and exits through a previously made sclerotomy. The other end of the suture is then externalized through the adjacent scleral incision. The needle is subsequently cut, and the two ends of the suture are tied extraocularly over the sclera and trimmed and the knot internalized. The procedure can also be repeated to address the size of iridodialysis, and all sclerotomies are sutured closed.

2.4.6 Traumatic Aniridia

Complete avulsion of the iris may occur in open globe trauma mostly due to a severe blunt trauma but may less frequently occur secondary to penetrating trauma [10]. The avulsed iris may be found retracted in the anterior chamber, occluding the angle, underneath the conjunctiva after escaping through a penetrating wound, or not be found inside or around the eye. Traumatic aniridia may occur alongside other ocular injuries, including lens subluxation/dislocation, anterior chamber angle damage, late PAS formation, and glaucoma (Fig. 2.7).

Correction of traumatic aniridia depends on whether cataract extraction or lensectomy will be undertaken. If no lens surgery is planned, the use of opaque, iris-print contact lenses is a suitable option. Surgical correction of traumatic aniridia usually involves the placement of an aniridia or a black diaphragm lens after lensectomy or cataract extraction in the sulcus, with the lens haptics placed in the bag or in the sulcus. These lenses may also be sulcus sutured or glued. Although the use of these lenses effectively reduces glare and improves cosmetic appearance, complications such as corneal decompensation, glaucoma, and decentration are commonly encountered [11]. Many other types of prosthetic iris devices (PIDs) are available, including iris-lens diaphragm PIDs, endocapsular capsular tension ring (CTR)-based PIDs, and customized artificial irides [12].

Tattooing of the mid-corneal stroma is a less popular option and, although can eliminate visual disturbances associated with traumatic aniridia, often has a poor cosmetic appearance, and eye color cannot be made to match that of the contralateral iris. It is usually reserved for blind eyes for cosmetic purposes and is rarely indicated in eyes with good visual potential or for elimination of glare symptoms.

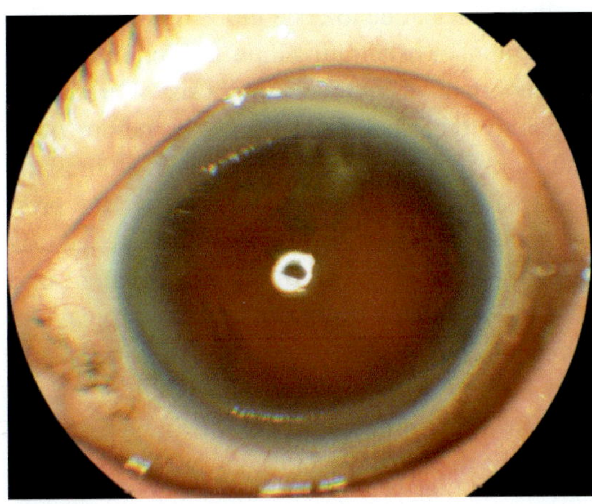

Fig. 2.7 Traumatic aniridia

2.4.7 Traumatic Ciliary Body Injury

Traumatic ciliary body injury can occur as a result of an open or closed globe injury and may result in iridocyclitis, traumatic hypotony, ciliary body detachment, ciliary body damage, or cyclodialysis cleft. It can also be associated with a range of other ocular injuries, including trauma to the corneoscleral shell, crystalline lens, iris, and/or posterior segment structures.

Ocular hypotony is often thought of as an intraocular pressure (IOP) less than 6.5 mmHg [13]. However, many of the complications of hypotony often do not manifest until the IOP is 4–5 mmHg or less [14]. Complications of ocular hypotony include reduced visual acuity, corneal edema and striae, shallow anterior chamber, cataract formation, choroidal effusion or hemorrhage, exudative retinal detachment (ERD), hypotony maculopathy, optic disk edema, and, eventually, phthisis bulbi [15–17].

The pathophysiology of traumatic hypotony is not completely understood and may at times be difficult to precisely determine. However, traumatic hypotony can generally result secondary to an imbalance between aqueous humor production and filtration and may be transient or persistent [13, 18, 19]. Excessive aqueous drainage can occur secondary to wound leak, ciliary body detachment, or cyclodialysis cleft, while reduced aqueous production may occur in cases of intraocular inflammation/iridocyclitis or ciliary body damage [19].

Wound leak due to open globe injuries secondary to blunt or penetrating injuries is common. It is an important differential diagnosis of traumatic hypotony that should be ruled out before other causes of hypotony are considered. A fluorescein strip Seidel test can be used to confirm the presence of a leak when the source of a presumed leak could not be easily identified. Management of a wound leak involves prompt, timely surgical closure of the wound to restore globe integrity, reverse hypotony, and minimize the risk of endophthalmitis. However, minimally leaking or self-sealing small full-thickness wounds may be managed conservatively with pressure patching or bandage contact lens placement, in addition to topical administration of aqueous suppressants, such as carbonic anhydrase inhibitors (CAIs) and β-blockers. Surgical closure of lacerations that are located far posteriorly (i.e., posterior to the equator) is difficult, and conservative, watchful management should be considered.

When an open globe is ruled out and no wound leak is presumed to be present, other potential causes of hypotony, such as cyclodialysis cleft and ciliary body detachment, should be considered. Traumatic ciliary body detachment usually occurs together with choroidal detachment (ciliochoroidal detachment) and is commonly associated with hypotony, breakdown of the blood-ocular barrier, and iridocyclitis. It may also coexist with a cyclodialysis cleft. Ciliochoroidal detachment is thought to reduce aqueous humor production. However, the reduction in aqueous outflow maybe attributed to concurrent iridocyclitis rather than ciliary body detachment per se [19]. The diagnosis can be made by observation of anterior choroidal detachment using binocular indirect ophthalmoscopy, B-scan ultrasonography, or ultrasound biomicroscopy (UBM). UBM can also precisely determine if a concurrent cyclodialysis cleft exists (Fig. 2.8). Treatment of ciliochoroidal detachment involves:

- Topical and systemic corticosteroids to treat concurrent iridocyclitis.
- Topical cycloplegic agents (e.g., 1 % atropine two to three times daily).
- Systemic carbonic anhydrase inhibitors (CAIs) may help improve suprachoroidal fluid absorption [19].
- Surgical treatment if no response to medical regimen for 3–4 weeks, with flat anterior chamber and/or PAS formation.

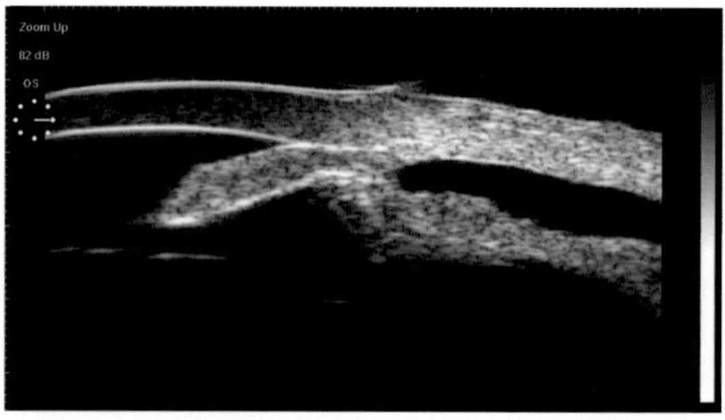

Fig. 2.8 Cyclodialysis cleft

Surgical treatment of a ciliochoroidal detachment by means of supraciliary/suprachoroidal fluid drainage is achieved by creating a fornix-based conjunctival flap, followed by the dissection of a partial-thickness scleral flap extending over the supraciliary and the suprachoroidal spaces [20]. A stab incision is then made into the supraciliary space, and fluid is subsequently drained. Multiple incisions are usually made. The ciliary body is sutured to the scleral spur using a permanent 10–0 polypropylene or nylon suture, if a cyclodialysis cleft is also identified preoperatively.

A cyclodialysis cleft typically results from a closed globe injury caused by significant blunt shear force trauma and represents disruption of the insertion of meridional ciliary muscle fibers into the scleral spur [21]. The cleft results in the creation of an abnormal aqueous humor drainage pathway into the suprachoroidal space causing hypotony. Cyclodialysis clefts are commonly associated with iridocyclitis and aqueous flare, which may hinder accurate measurement of aqueous production [19]. The earlier concept attributing hypotony associated with cyclodialysis clefts to reduced aqueous humor production is challenged, since eyes with a cyclodialysis cleft and no aqueous flare were shown to have normal aqueous outflow as measured by fluorophotometry [22]. Sudden closure of cyclodialysis clefts may cause a rapid, severe rise in intraocular pressure (IOP) which needs to be observed closely in the acute postoperative period [23]. However, a cleft may reopen upon using miotic agents, and IOP may again fall to hypotonous levels [24].

Clinical diagnosis of cyclodialysis clefts is challenging, given the softness of the eye, associated corneal edema, and occasionally trauma hyphema, which may render gonioscopy very difficult [22, 25]. Ultrasound biomicroscopy (UBM) and anterior segment optical coherence tomography (AS-OCT) have therefore been increasingly utilized in the diagnosis of this condition. Sometimes an occult cleft may be present, and dynamic testing with indentation to open a cleft while imaging a cleft or viewing through a gonioprism is needed to identify the presence and extent of a cleft. Identifying the location and extent of the cleft is crucial to formulating a management plan, since multiple clefts may be present, and overlooking one of them may warrant a secondary therapeutic intervention [25].

Small clefts (less than 2–3 h) may respond to a 6–8-week course of cycloplegic-mydriatic agents (e.g., 1 % atropine twice daily), since cycloplegia relaxes the ciliary muscle, allowing its apposition to the sclera [15, 21, 23]. Reduction or elimination of corticosteroids, when feasible, may also induce an inflammatory reaction that may facilitate ciliary muscle adhesion to the sclera [26].

When pharmacologic treatment fails to achieve closure of the cyclodialysis cleft, a number of minimally invasive, nonsurgical procedures can be tried, including argon and diode laser photocoagulation, transscleral diathermy, and cryotherapy [25–33]. These treatments generate inflammation that may help scar the cleft closed. Although a reemergence of interest in some of these techniques exists, strong evidence of their safety, efficacy, and reproducibility is lacking [25].

Surgical repair is the treatment modality of choice for medium to large-sized clefts after initial less invasive modalities have elicited an insufficient response [34]. Many surgical techniques have been developed to achieve cyclodialysis cleft closure. A commonly used technique involves marking of the preoperatively determined cleft location; creation of peritomy; cutting of a partial-thickness scleral flap, followed by passing a needle with 9–0 or 10–0 polypropylene (Prolene) or nylon suture through the scleral bed to engage; and reattachment of the ciliary body to the sclera to surgically close the cleft (Fig. 2.9).

2.4.8 Traumatic Lens Injury

Mechanical ocular trauma can damage the crystalline lens by inducing loss of transparency (cataract), loss of position (subluxation, dislocation, or extrusion), or both (Fig. 2.10a, b). Traumatic cataract can result secondary to both blunt and penetrating mechanical ocular injuries

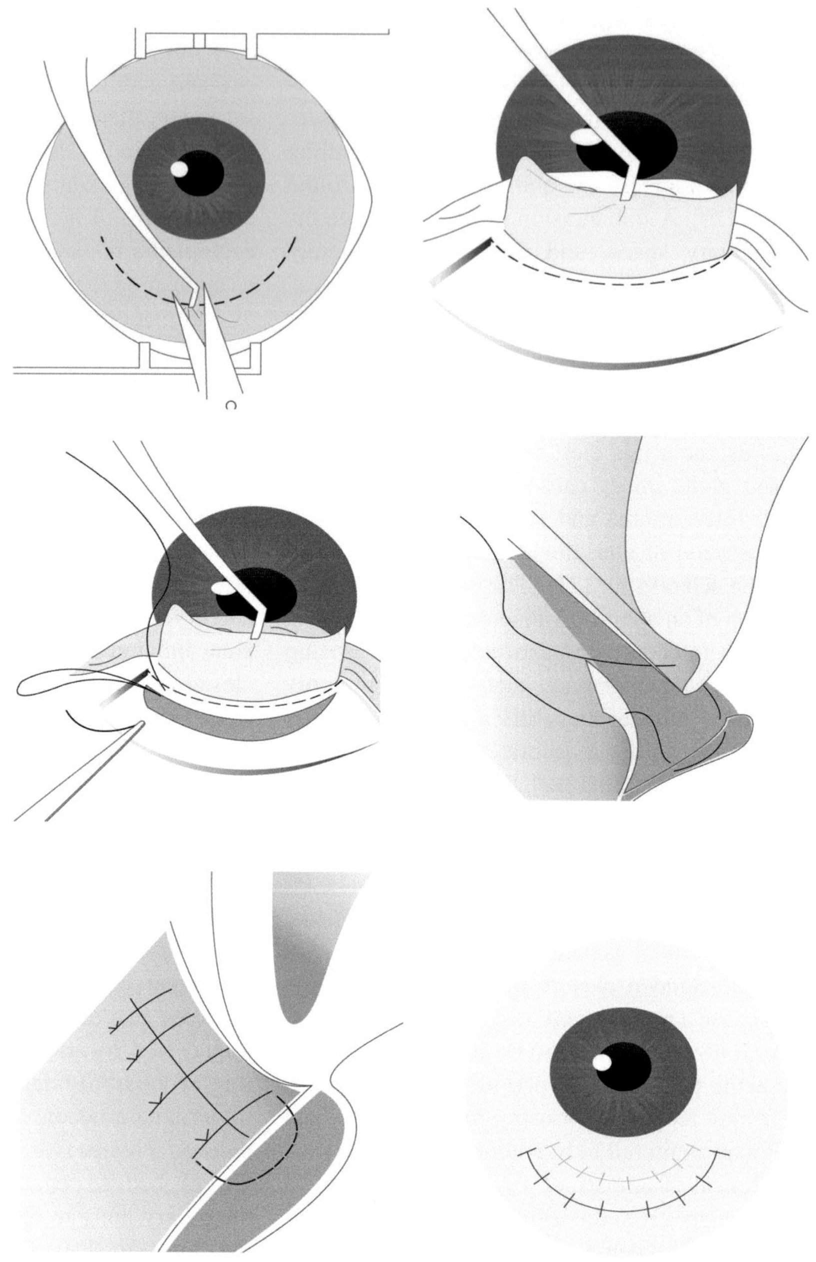

Fig. 2.9 Surgical repair of cyclodialysis cleft

and demographically affects patients of all ages, with 53 % of patients falling between 7 and 30 years of age [35]. Male patients are four times more often affected than are female patients [35]. Definitive treatment of traumatic cataract or lens subluxation/dislocation, like that of all other forms of crystalline lens pathology, is surgical.

Although surgical extraction of age-related cataract is relatively simple and carries a great success rate, surgical treatment of traumatic cataract can be more technically challenging, and outcomes are generally less favorable depending on the amount and type of trauma. This is mainly due to:

- Reduced visibility: with cloudy media (corneal laceration, intense inflammatory reaction in the anterior chamber, hyphema, intraocular foreign body)

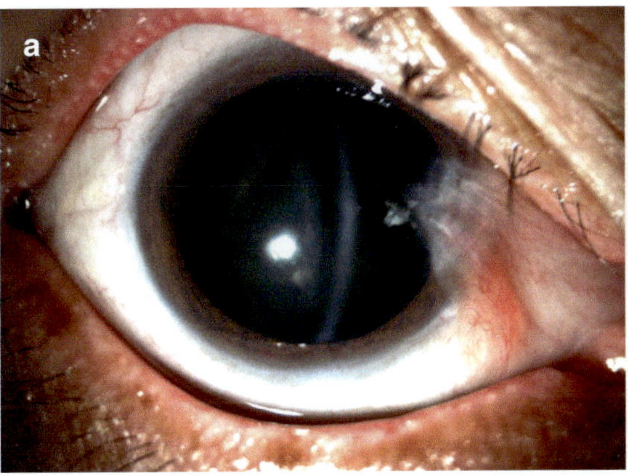

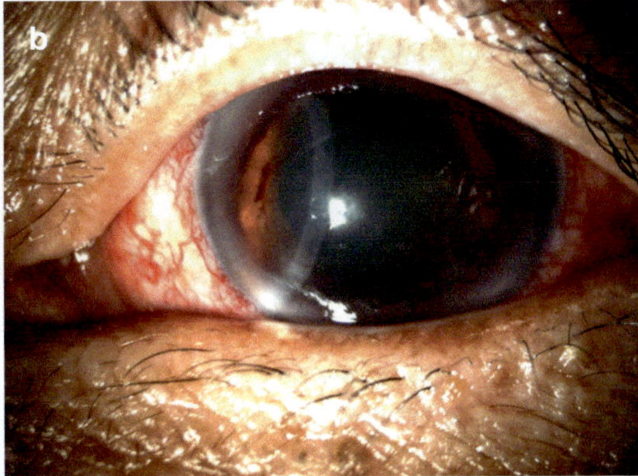

Fig. 2.10 (**a**) Traumatic lens subluxation and (**b**) traumatic lens dislocation into the anterior chamber

- Disruption of globe integrity in open globe injuries
- Difficult wound construction: due to loss of anterior chamber volume and uveal prolapse
- Difficult capsulorhexis: traumatic capsular injury, loss of contrast due to vitreous hemorrhage, loose zonular support, and poor view with corneal edema
- Difficult nucleus disassembly: loose zonular support, lens subluxation, and lens dislocation
- Concomitant injury to other anterior segment structures: poor pupil dilation, iris laceration, and iridodialysis
- Vitreous prolapse: either preoperatively or as an intraoperative complication
- Required use of often unfamiliar devices/instrumentation: iris retractors, capsular tension rings, vitrectomy instrumentation, and iris-fixated or scleral-fixated intraocular lenses (IOLs)

Preoperative evaluation of traumatic cataract should therefore aim at determining:

- Globe integrity status: open globe vs. closed globe injury. Determining if there is a corneal, limbal, or scleral laceration (or any combination of these) that must be addressed before management of the traumatic cataract is a critically important step in the evaluation of these cases. Care must be taken to avoid overlooking occult scleral lacerations that may be obscured by subconjunctival hemorrhage or rectus muscle insertions, especially in the presence of conjunctival lacerations.
- Visual significance of cataract: this can be difficult to determine in the presence of cloudy media (cornea, anterior chamber, or vitreous) or retinal pathology. Lens opacities that are off the visual axis generally induce less vision loss than do more central opacities.
- Intraocular pressure in closed globe injuries.
- Anterior chamber status: lost volume, fibrin, hyphema, lens material, or vitreous prolapse.
- Anterior capsule: intact vs. injured/torn.
- Lens clarity: is the lens clear or cataractous (total, membranous, cortical, white soft, or rosette shaped)? Is a Vossius ring present?
- Lens location: in place, anteriorly dislocated in the anterior chamber, posteriorly dislocated in the vitreous cavity, or extruded extraocularly. Posteriorly dislocated crystalline lenses may be surgically treated by pars plana vitrectomy and lens fragmentation.
- Lens integrity: is the lens fragmented or one piece? Has the lens capsule been violated?
- Posterior capsule integrity. This is very important in surgical planning since cases in which the posterior capsule is breached are generally managed with pars plana lensectomy and vitrectomy. If preoperative determination of posterior capsule integrity is not possible, intraoperative assessment under the surgical microscope can sometimes be achieved.
- Zonular support: is the lens held firmly in place or is there iridodonesis/phacodonesis?

Location of weak zonular support should be determined when possible.

- Status of the iris, angle, and ciliary body: iris laceration, iridodialysis, angle recession, or cyclodialysis.
- The presence of an intraocular foreign body (IOFB) or an intralenticular foreign body.
- Pupil reaction/dilation.
- Retina/vitreous status: vitreous prolapse, vitreous hemorrhage, retinal breaks, retinal hemorrhages, or retinal detachment. If adequate fundus examination cannot be attained, diagnostic B-scan ultrasonography should be performed with extreme care if loss of globe integrity is a concern.

Diagnostic B-scan ultrasonography, computed tomography (CT) scan, and newer imaging technologies such as Scheimpflug imaging can be used in cases in which the status of the lens, posterior capsule integrity, or the presence of an intralenticular foreign body (Fig. 2.11) cannot be determined by slit lamp biomicroscopy due to corneal laceration, corneal edema, anterior chamber fibrin, hyphema, or ineffective pupil dilation [36–39], although their diagnostic accuracy is questioned and certain artifacts can be misleading [40, 41].

2.4.8.1 Timing of Surgery

Primary cataract surgery to address traumatic cataract and/or lens subluxation/dislocation has certain advantages over secondary surgery, including:

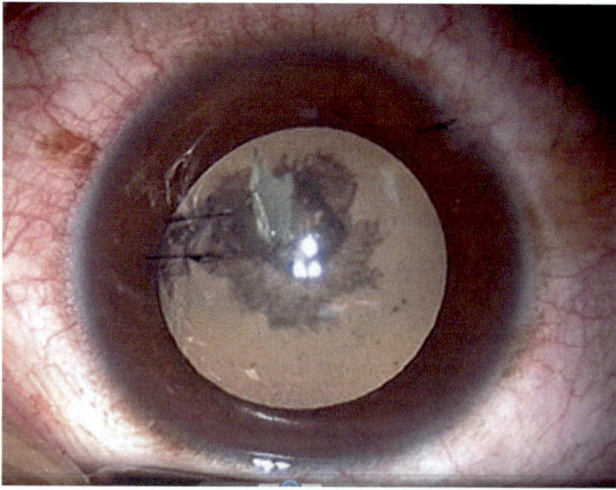

Fig. 2.11 Intralenticular foreign body

- Faster visual rehabilitation: particularly in children in whom development of amblyopia is a major concern and in patients whose occupations require faster regain of visual acuity
- Earlier elimination of lens-induced inflammation: particularly when the anterior lens capsule has been breached
- Avoidance or definitive treatment of lens-induced intraocular pressure (IOP) elevation or glaucomas including phacomorphic, phacoanaphylactic, lens particle, or lens subluxation/dislocation-associated (e.g., pupillary block) glaucomas
- Elimination of refractive fluctuations resulting from the instability of subluxated lenses
- Allowing prompt examination of, or future surgical intervention involving, the posterior segment
- Elimination of undue vitreous traction on the retina when vitreous prolapse or traction is present that may lead to a retinal detachment

However, surgery may be deferred until certain surgeon-related or center-related factors are addressed (e.g., availability of a more experienced surgeon able to undertake technically challenging techniques, trained support personnel, or special instrumentation that may not be available to the surgeon in emergent surgeries that are performed outside normal working hours such as vitrectomy, capsular tension rings, or special IOLs). Surgery is also better deferred if the cataract is presumed to be visually insignificant, particularly in the absence of coexisting ocular injuries requiring surgery. However, traumatic cataracts can be stationary or progressive (particularly in the presence of an intralenticular foreign body due to siderosis) [42, 43], and regular follow-up is required to rule out progression of traumatic cataracts initially considered visually insignificant.

2.4.8.2 Type of Surgery/Surgical Technique

Primary closure of globe lacerations (corneal, limbal, scleral, or corneoscleral), when present, is the first step in the management of traumatic cataract, since a formed globe is necessary for safe cataract removal. Constructing a separate incision for the removal of cataract (clear corneal, limbal, scleral, or pars plana) is preferred to utilizing the existing traumatic corneal wound to avoid inflicting damage to the endothelium or inducing Descemet's detachment [44]. Liberal use of ophthalmic viscoelastic devices (OVDs) or the use of an anterior chamber maintainer should be employed to keep the globe formed at all times and to avoid potentially devastating complications such as suprachoroidal hemorrhage (SCH). The anterior chamber should be washed to remove hyphema to improve the view, and any floating lens particles should be removed. Anterior chamber vitrectomy should also be performed when vitreous strands are visible anterior to the crystalline lens plane. The pupil should be dilated using iris retractors or pupil-dilating (e.g., Malyugin) rings if the pupil is not readily and sufficiently dilated, and capsular staining should be considered to improve the view for capsulorhexis.

Important factors to consider when determining the method of cataract removal are:

1. Amount of zonular support
2. Posterior capsule integrity
3. Density of the cataract
4. View of the cataract

In cases in which zonular support is deemed to be sufficient for safe removal of the cataract through an anterior (limbal) approach, cataract can be removed using manual extracapsular cataract extraction (ECCE), phacoemulsification, or vitrectomy. Capsulorhexis can be challenging in the traumatic cataract. Minimal downward pressure on the lens and compression of the lens should be carried out using a pair of capsulorhexis (e.g., Utrata) forceps or a cystotome needle in order to avoid further weakening of the zonules. The capsulorhexis should start away from the presumed area of zonular weakness. Partial capsulorhexis may be done, followed by, when necessary, insertion of capsule retractors to support the area of zonular loss, before capsulorhexis is safely completed. Capsular tension rings or ring segments can be used either after performing capsulorhexis or prior to nuclear disassembly in phacoemulsification. Capsular microscissors (which insert through a paracentesis) may be used if the anterior capsule is torn and the direction of tear does not allow safe redirection of the capsular flap to achieve a continuous, curvilinear capsulorhexis to avoid extension of the anterior capsule tear. Capsular staining using trypan blue dye under an air bubble should be used in traumatic cataracts where adequate visibility of the capsule cannot be achieved, due to the lack of a contrasting red reflex due to either a hard cataract, vitreous hemorrhage, or milky white traumatic cataract.

Phacoemulsification (with low vacuum and aspiration settings to avoid anterior chamber size fluctuation and prevent further zonular damage) [45] is the preferred technique when the posterior capsule is intact and adequate zonular support is present due to its less traumatic nature and faster visual recovery. Manual ECCE or slow-motion phacoemulsification can be carefully attempted if the status of the posterior capsule cannot be precisely determine in the presence of good zonular support or in the presence of a small posterior capsule rent with no vitreous prolapse. If the chamber is deep enough, supracapsular cataract extraction is also a good approach to remove the lens since this approach, with the partial prolapse of the cataract in the iris plane for phacoemulsification, reduces zonular stress with the lens being fractured outside the capsular bag.

The surgeon needs to be ready to switch to vitrectomy if vitreous prolapse is detected. Posterior-assisted levitation (PAL) using a 1-mm spatula inserted through a pars plana sclerotomy created by a microvitreoretinal (MVR) blade 3.5-mm posterior to the limbus to lift the posterior capsule-lens complex upward and resume phacoemulsification of remaining nuclear fragments may be attempted by experienced surgeons when a rent in the posterior capsule is inadvertently brought about or becomes evident or when further zonular damage is inflicted during nuclear fragmentation [46]. This technique can also be planned preoperatively in subluxated lenses thought to not be adequately fixable using capsular tension rings. Viscoelastic agents should be liberally used to return into the vitreous cavity any vitreous strands attached to the posterior capsule or prolapsing into the bag or anterior chamber if this technique is used. However, the technique is technically challenging and carries a risk of significant complications such as nuclear drop and retinal detachment. Intracapsular cataract extraction (ICCE), while can be employed in cases of significantly severed zonular support, requires the creation of a large incision and carries a high risk of suprachoroidal hemorrhage (SCH) [44].

In the presence of vitreous prolapse or a large rent in the posterior capsule, or if there is an indication of a posterior segment surgery at the time of cataract extraction, pars plana lensectomy/vitrectomy (PPLV), with the possible aid of phacofragmentation in hard nuclei, is the procedure of choice [44]. Lens removal using the vitrector has the advantage of utilizing a small incision and minimizing the risk of suprachoroidal hemorrhage (SCH). The pars plana approach, while requires special expertise and equipment, is preferred to corneal or limbal approaches when vitrectomy is planned, since it maintains corneal clarity and achieves a more complete vitrectomy behind the iris plane [44].

Age of the traumatic cataract patient is also an important determinant of the surgical technique to be employed. In young children, performing primary posterior capsulotomy and anterior vitrectomy is indicated due to the high rate of posterior capsule opacification [47, 48]. Anterior and posterior lens capsules are very elastic in young children, and standard continuous curvilinear capsulorhexis (CCC) is technically challenging. Vitrectorhexis is gaining popularity as an equally effective alternative to anterior and posterior CCC in children, with the added benefit of being faster, more predictable, and reproducible and requiring only a short learning curve [49–51]. The authors prefer using the vitrectomy system for cutting the lens matter through a limbal incision with the aid of an anterior chamber maintainer over the older irrigation/aspiration techniques for soft pediatric cataracts. A separate pars plana port is subsequently created for posterior vitrectorhexis and limited anterior vitrectomy, although suturing the sclerotomy site may be required, even with the use of 23-gauge and 25-gauge vitrectomy systems [49].

The age also determines the vitrectomy settings to be used when cutting the nuclear matter utilizing the vitrectomy system is planned. In children and young adults, using only aspiration without cutting usually suffices, with more cutting required with older patients and harder cataracts.

2.4.8.3 Intraocular Lens (IOL) Implantation

Preservation of anterior and/or posterior capsular support to allow in-the-bag or in-sulcus implantation of IOLs is an important goal of surgery in most traumatic cataract. However, achieving adequate capsular support is not always feasible, especially when the degree of zonular loss is significant or when pars plana lensectomy/vitrectomy is employed, and in some complex cases, it may be better to leave a patient aphakic and take a staged approach for refractive purposes.

When enough anterior and posterior capsular support permissive of in-the-bag IOL implantation is present, it is best to proceed with in-the-bag implantation, since the IOL-capsular bag complex is more resilient and resistant to subsequent trauma [52]. Three-piece foldable IOLs are preferred over single-piece IOLs since three-piece lenses provide more tensile strength, can provide enough support in mild degrees of zonular loss when implanted in the bag, and may afford better resistance to capsular phimosis [53–55]. Moreover, the optic of a three-piece lens can be captured in the bag with placement of the haptics in the sulcus to provide additional tensile support.

Sulcus implantation of a three-piece foldable IOL is indicated when the capsular support available is not enough to permit in-the-bag implantation of the IOL or anterior optic capture. Viscoelastic agents should be injected in the ciliary sulcus between the iris and the remaining capsular support in order to insure proper placement of the IOL optic and haptics in the sulcus. Central polishing or removal of the capsular support tissue is recommended in such cases [56].

If no enough capsular support permissive of IOL implantation in the bag or in sulcus or when such positioning may result in a significant IOL tilt with or without the use of capsular tension rings, the use of an angle-supported anterior chamber IOL, sulcus-sutured or glued posterior chamber IOL, or iris-fixated IOL is indicated following anterior vitrectomy. The visual outcome achieved using these techniques is generally comparable [57].

Angle-supported anterior chamber IOLs are implanted in close proximity to the posterior corneal surface. Therefore, they have the potential for inducing corneal decompensation and precipitating pseudophakic bullous keratopathy (PBK), especially when the older model is used [58, 59]. It is important that the haptics are well seated in the angle to minimize PAS and effects on the cornea. These types of IOLs in younger patients or in patients in whom the axial length and/or anterior chamber depth (ACD) is relatively small may have greater long-term complications.

Various techniques for fixating IOLs to the ciliary sulcus have been described. Sutured scleral fixation of IOLs with specialized haptics harboring suture eyelets can be achieved using double-armed permanent 8-0 or 9-0 polypropylene sutures and long straight or curved hollow needles (Fig. 2.12a–h) [57]. Most techniques utilize scleral flaps, tunnels, or grooves to provide access to the ciliary sulcus, bury the knots, and guard against suture erosion/exposure. However, difficult centration, IOL tilt, and rotational and anteroposterior instability are potential pitfalls of sulcus-sutured IOLs and may warrant secondary surgical intervention. A peripheral iridectomy using the vitrectomy system is recommended to prevent pupillary block glaucoma. This is achieved by introducing the vitrector into the anterior chamber at the 12 or 9 o'clock position

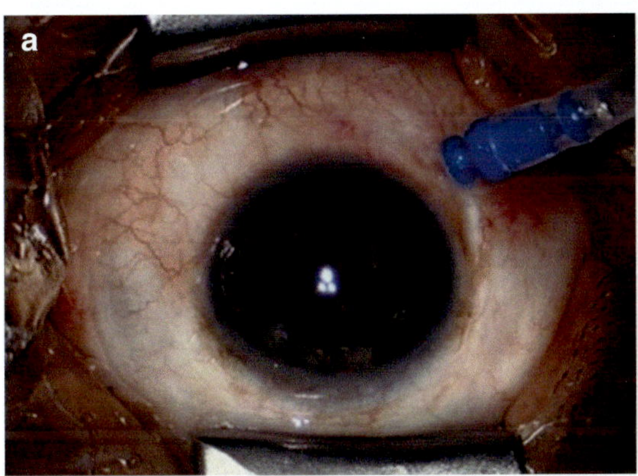

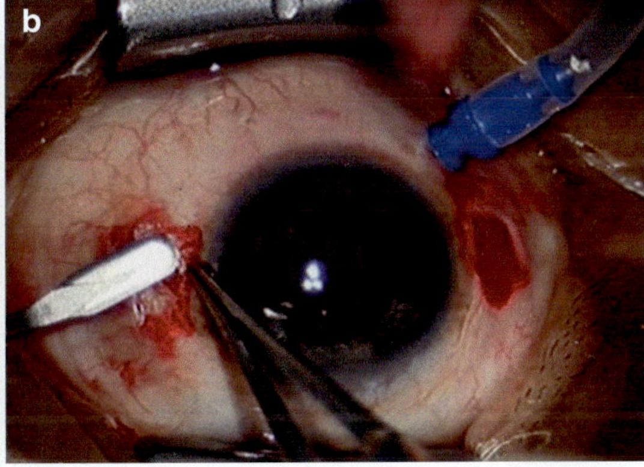

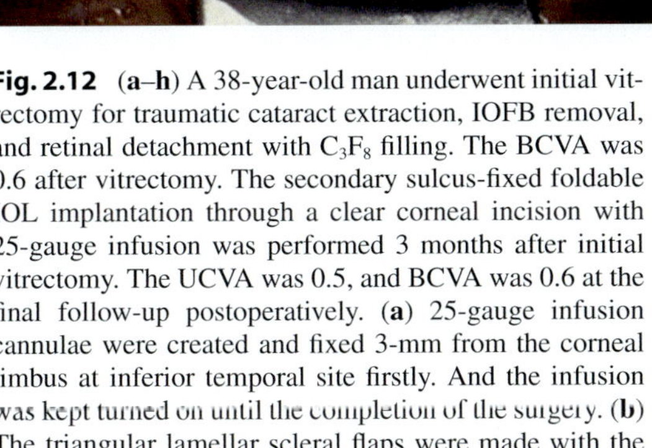

Fig. 2.12 (**a**–**h**) A 38-year-old man underwent initial vitrectomy for traumatic cataract extraction, IOFB removal, and retinal detachment with C_3F_8 filling. The BCVA was 0.6 after vitrectomy. The secondary sulcus-fixed foldable IOL implantation through a clear corneal incision with 25-gauge infusion was performed 3 months after initial vitrectomy. The UCVA was 0.5, and BCVA was 0.6 at the final follow-up postoperatively. (**a**) 25-gauge infusion cannulae were created and fixed 3-mm from the corneal limbus at inferior temporal site firstly. And the infusion was kept turned on until the completion of the surgery. (**b**) The triangular lamellar scleral flaps were made with the corneal limbus as base (black arrow) at 3 and 9 o'clock, respectively, for protecting the IOL suture. (**c**) The suture needle (10–0 polypropylene) entered the eye under the sclera flap at 9 o'clock and was relayed into a 1-mL syringe needle in the posterior chamber which entered the eye at 3 o'clock. (**d**) A 3.0-mm clear corneal incision was made, and the 10–0 polypropylene suture was pulled out through the incision. (**e**) The foldable lens was put in the IOL injector and was pushed until the front haptic just exposed from the cartridge. Then the front haptic was tied by 10–0 polypropylene for preparing fixation. (**f**) The foldable lens was pushed into the posterior chamber with the posterior haptic left out of the incision. (**g**) The posterior haptic was tied by 10–0 polypropylene for preparing fixation. (**h**) The foldable IOL was fixed by suturing in the sulcus with a well-centered position

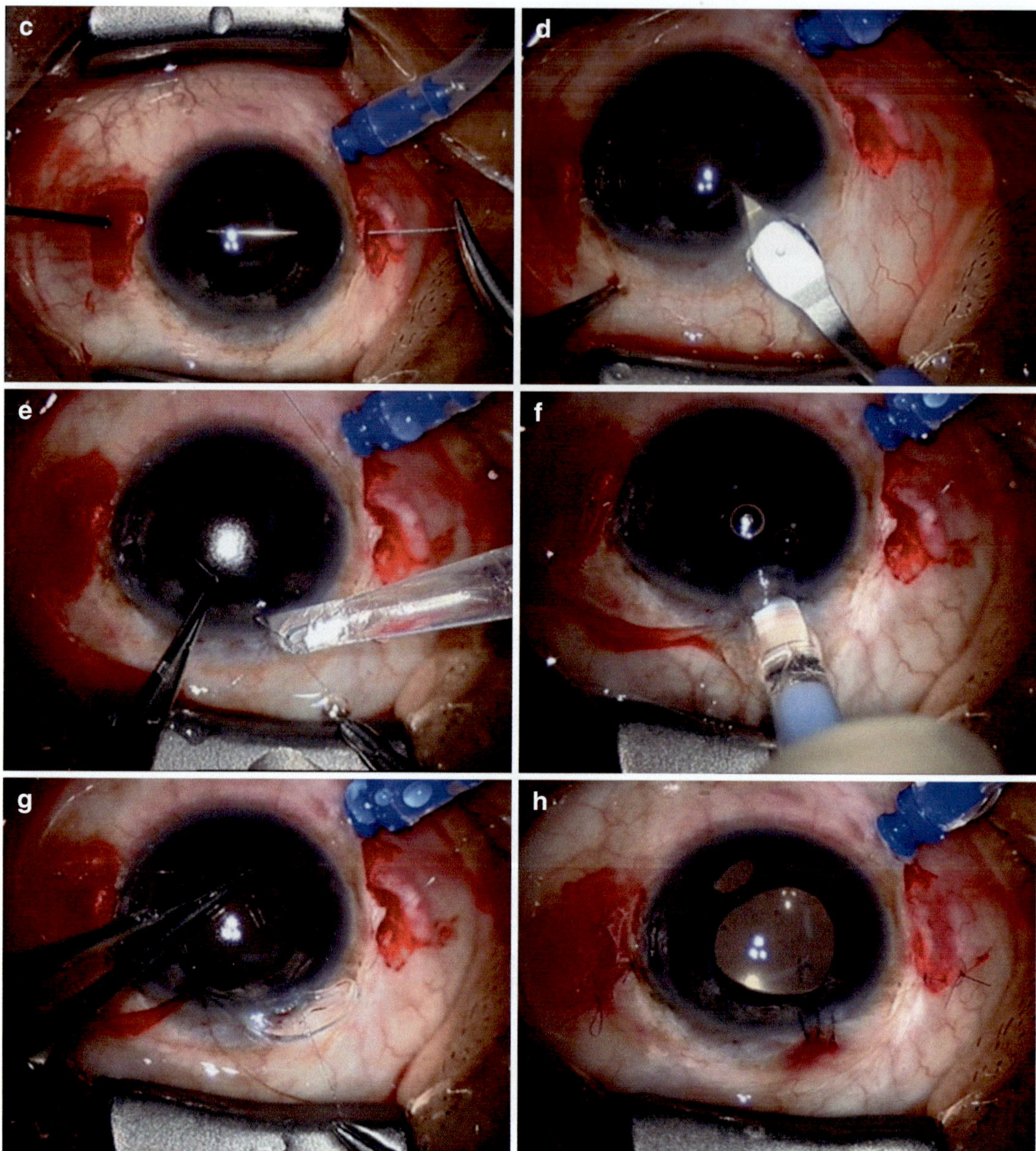

Fig. 2.12 (continued)

with the port facing down, cutting rate initially set to zero, and an aspiration pressure of 300 mmHg. Once occlusion is achieved, the cutting speed is carefully increased until a full, patent iridectomy is made. In cases of traumatic coexisting aniridia, a black diaphragm tinted IOL (Fig. 2.13) may be sutured to the sulcus [60].

Sutureless sulcus fixation of IOLs can be achieved with the utility of scleral flaps, limbus parallel tunnels, or both [57]. Sulcus-glued IOLs (Fig. 2.14) are becoming exceedingly popular and are thought to have better stability and fewer postoperative complications than do sulcus-sutured IOLs [61–65]. The technique of the procedure involves insertion of an infusion cannula or an anterior chamber maintainer, creation of two limbal-based, partial-thickness scleral flaps 180° apart, and performing two sclerotomies underneath the flaps 1.5-mm from the limbus [66]. This is followed by limited pars plana or

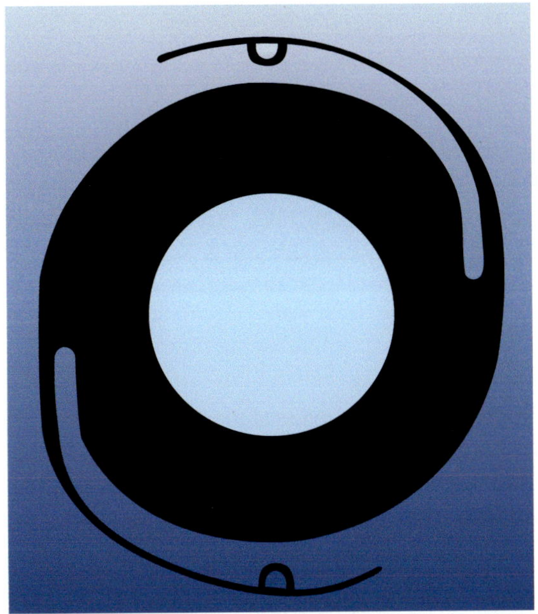

Fig. 2.13 A black diaphragm tinted IOL

limbal anterior vitrectomy to remove all vitreous strands in the anterior chamber, anterior vitreous cavity, and sclerotomy sites. Two scleral tunnels are then created in the edge of the scleral bed underlying the flaps adjacent and parallel to the limbus and following the curvature of the IOL haptics. These tunnels are created in such a way to allow tucking of the IOL haptics once externalized. The IOL is then introduced through a limbal-based incision and the two haptics externalized through the sclerotomies and tucked into the limbal scleral tunnels. Proper IOL centration is ensured by adjusting the tucked length of each haptic. Fibrin glue is then applied over the haptics underneath the scleral flaps which are subsequently repositioned. The infusion cannula or the anterior chamber maintainer is then removed, and the overlying conjunctiva is closed using the same glue. A glued aniridia IOL may also be used in cases of coexisting aniridia [67].

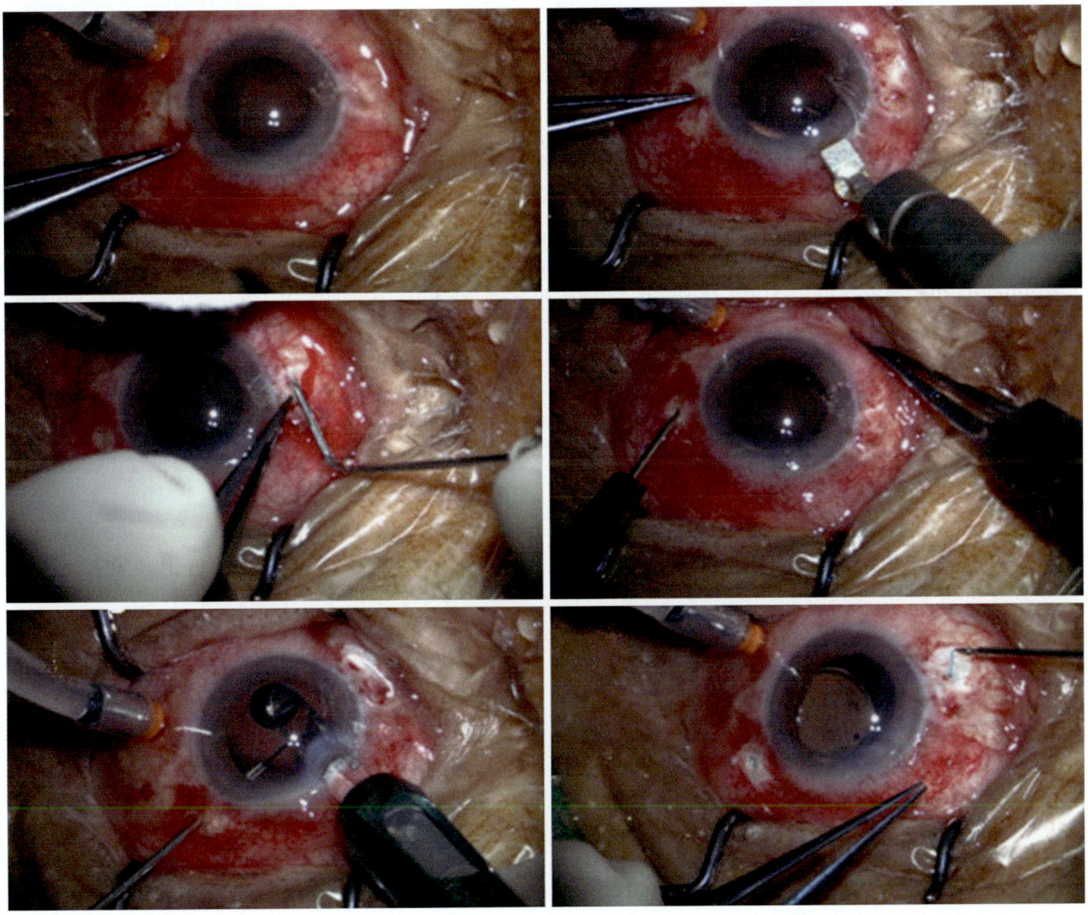

Fig. 2.14 Sulcus-glued IOLs

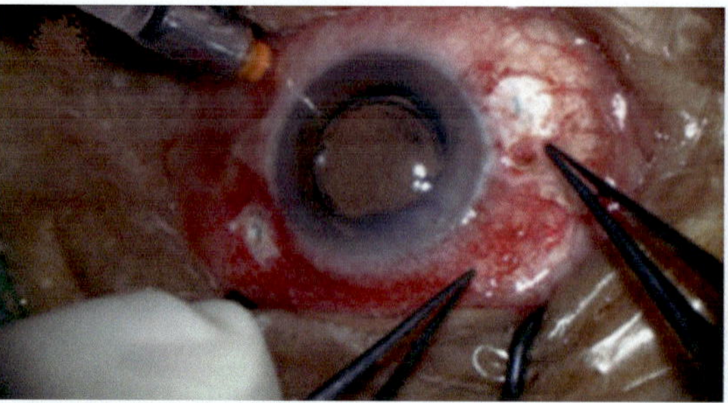
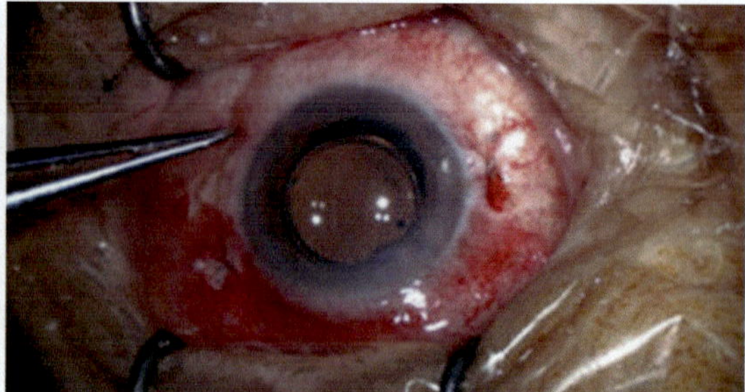

Fig. 2.14 (continued)

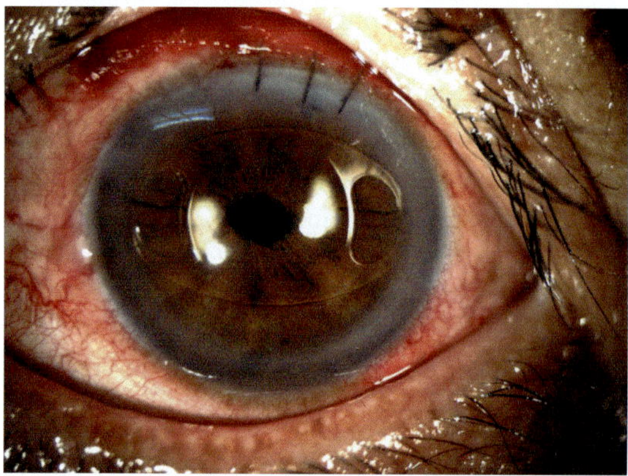

Fig. 2.15 Iris-claw lenses

Iris-claw lenses (e.g., Artisan/Verisyse "rigid" and Artiflex "foldable" lenses, Ophtec BV, Groningen, the Netherlands) are popular phakic IOLs used in refractive surgery in patients with high degrees of ametropia (Fig. 2.15) [68–70]. They have, however, been widely used for the correction of aphakia in the absence of sufficient capsular support in adults and children [71–73]. The technique of implantation of iris-claw lenses entails creation of an appropriately sized clear corneal incision centered at the 12 o'clock position and two side ports aligned with the enclavation sites, injection of a miotic agent, filling the anterior chamber with a cohesive viscoelastic, and introduction of the lens into the anterior chamber through the main wound. The lens is then rotated 90° so that the iris claws are horizontally placed in line with the side ports. Iris enclavation of the lens claws is then achieved through the two side port incisions, where a knuckle of iris tissue is captured by the claws on either side of the lens. A peripheral iridectomy is then made at the 12 o'clock position using the vitrectomy system as explained above. Although iris-claw lenses are considered effective in achieving the desired refractive outcome, the relatively high rate of endothelial cell loss remains a major concern [71, 74]. The retro-enclavation of these lenses to the posterior surface of the iris in aphakic eyes has thus become an attractive alternative to anterior iris enclavation, achieving a comparable refractive outcome and inducing less endothelial cell loss [75–77]. Other complications that could result from iris-claw lens implantation include trauma to the iris vessels with subsequent intraocular bleeding, interference with pupillary dilation, dyscoria, and peripheral anterior synechiae formation [57, 78, 79].

Intraocular lens (IOL) power calculation poses a challenge in cases of traumatic cataract and/or lens subluxation or dislocation, since reliable biometry may be difficult to obtain on the traumatized eye. However, biometry from the contralateral eye may be used in such cases [35, 56, 80]. IOL power is generally reduced as the lens is implanted further anteriorly in the eye, with sulcus-fixated and iris-enclaved/angle-supported lens power reduced a half and a full diopter than is in-the-bag lens power, respectively.

Timing of IOL implantation in traumatic cataract and/or lens subluxation/dislocation has been a controversial issue [44]. Several studies demonstrated favorable results of primary IOL implantation performed at the time of initial reconstruction, with many advocating such strategy [35, 56, 80, 81]. However, complications such as fibrinous uveitis, synechia formation, pupillary capture, retinal detachment, and other posterior segment complications have been associated with primary IOL implantation in these cases [44, 82–85]. Moreover, primary IOL implantation is sometimes deferred in pediatric patients due to sizing and refractive factors (e.g., myopic shift) [86], although it may guard against the development of amblyopia [87], and is advocated by some as early as 8 months of age [88], especially in children in whom contact lens wear is not suitable. In general, primary IOL implantation is better avoided in the following conditions [44]:

- Children younger than 1 year of age
- Highly myopic patients who may not need refractive correction for aphakia
- Large corneal lacerations with significant damage to the corneal endothelium or in cases in which a corneal transplant might be planned in the future
- Scleral lacerations
- High risk of endophthalmitis
- Traumatic aniridia/significant iris damage
- Cyclodialysis or angle recession
- Retinal detachment
- Significant posterior segment trauma or inability to assess degree of posterior segment involvement
- High likelihood of proliferative vitreoretinopathy (PVR)

2.4.9 Traumatic Glaucoma

Traumatic glaucoma is a collective term that encompasses a myriad of different disease processes that occur following ocular trauma secondary to variable pathophysiologic and reparative mechanisms whose common end result is chronic intraocular pressure (IOP) elevation and glaucomatous optic neuropathy. The management of this group of glaucoma is challenging, and complex surgical procedures to restore normal ocular anatomy and/or lower IOP are often necessary. The risk of developing glaucoma following blunt trauma was reported to be 19 % in one study [89], while it was found to be only 3 % following penetrating ocular trauma in another study [90]. Trauma is one of the most common causes of glaucoma in individuals younger than 30 years of age (35.9 %) [91], given the higher incidence of trauma in this age group (58 %) [92], particularly among males [93, 94].

Traumatic glaucoma can be classified according to the mechanism of trauma (blunt vs. penetrating), globe integrity (open globe vs. closed globe), onset of glaucoma following trauma (early onset vs. late onset), and state of the anterior chamber angle (open angle vs. angle closure). The classification scheme summarized in Fig. 2.16 takes all these parameters into consideration.

2.4.9.1 General Considerations for the Management of Traumatic Glaucoma

Since many cases of traumatic glaucoma involve disruption of normal ocular anatomy or are associated with conditions that are only surgically correctable such as cataract or retinal detachment, medical therapy alone is usually not sufficient to address these issues. However, topical and/or medical therapies are typically administered to lower IOP in cases of open-angle, closed globe traumatic glaucomas, in preparation for subsequent surgical intervention, or postoperatively.

Traditionally, topical β-blockers (e.g., timolol or levobunolol 0.5 %), α-2 adrenergic agonists (e.g., apraclonidine 0.5 % or brimonidine 0.15 %), and topical (e.g., dorzolamide 2 % or brinzolamide 1 %) and systemic (e.g., acetazolamide or methazolamide) carbonic anhydrase inhibitors (CAIs) have been used for these purposes. Prostaglandin analogs (PGAs) have theoretically been considered pro-inflammatory and have thus been avoided in types of glaucoma in which there is significant intraocular inflammation and/or a disruption in the blood-aqueous barrier, such as traumatic glaucomas. However, consensus to consider traumatic glaucomas, an absolute contraindication for the use of PGAs does not exist, and they have been safely and successfully used in the management of types of glaucoma in which intraocular inflammation is pronounced [95]. Cholinergic agents/miotics (e.g., pilocarpine) are

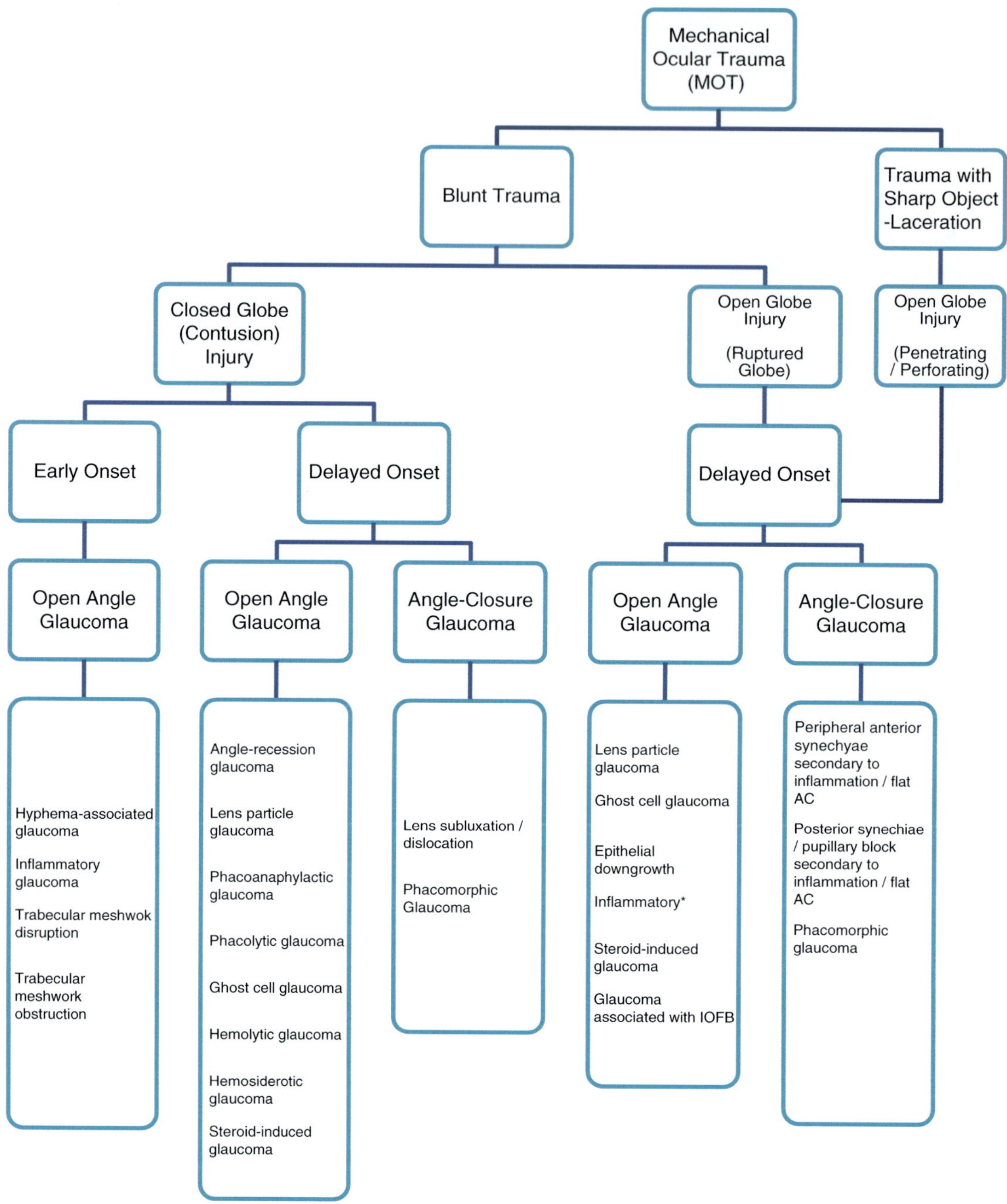

Fig. 2.16 Traumatic glaucoma (*can also be early onset)

better avoided in certain traumatic glaucomas, such as angle recession glaucoma, since they may paradoxically impair uveoscleral outflow when there is severe compromise to trabecular outflow, causing a net rise in IOP [96]. Moreover, miotics may increase vascular permeability and fibrin deposition in the setting of intraocular inflammation, may promote iridolenticular adhesions and seclusio pupillae, and can hinder thorough fundus examination [97].

Topical and systemic CAIs are avoided in patients with sickle cell disease or trait with high

IOP secondary to traumatic hyphema, since these drugs tend to acidify the aqueous humor and induce sickling of red blood cells (RBCs). If however necessary, systemic methazolamide may be safer than acetazolamide in this regard. Alpha-2 agonists are also better avoided in sickle cell disease or trait and in all patients younger than 3 years of age for the risk of apnea. Systemic hyperosmotic agents (e.g., mannitol) can induce hemoconcentration, acidosis, and sickling crisis in severely dehydrated patients with sickle cell disease or trait and are generally not recommended in these patients.

Cycloplegic agents (e.g., cyclopentolate 1 %) are used to reduce pain from ciliary muscle spasm, prevent the development of posterior synechiae, break newly formed synechiae, and facilitate posterior segment evaluation in traumatic hyphema and inflammatory glaucoma [95, 98]. Topical corticosteroid agents (e.g., prednisolone acetate) are used to reduce intraocular inflammation and may be of benefit in lowering the risk of rebleeding in traumatic hyphema [99]. Steroids should be tapered off as soon as signs of intraocular inflammation (anterior chamber cells and flare), fresh intraocular bleeding, photophobia, aching ocular pain, and ciliary injection resolve to reduce the possibility of steroid-induced glaucoma. Aspirin and systemic nonsteroidal anti-inflammatory medications are better avoided unless otherwise medically necessary and anticoagulation therapy discontinued after consultation with the appropriate specialist when intraocular bleeding is present. Mild, nonsedating systemic analgesics (e.g., acetaminophen) may be given when necessary.

Laser and surgical procedures used in specific types of traumatic glaucomas will be discussed in the respective sections.

2.4.9.2 Traumatic Hyphema-Associated Glaucoma

Hyphema is one of the most common causes of glaucoma secondary to mechanical ocular trauma. It commonly results from sports-related injuries [100], with males outnumbering women with a 3:1 ratio [101]. The main complications that may arise secondary to traumatic hyphema are:

- Elevated IOP
- Rebleeding
- Corneal blood staining
- Glaucomatous optic atrophy
- Posterior and/or peripheral anterior synechiae (PAS) formation

Initially, sudden transient rise in IOP when the eye sustains a blunt contusion injury can result in mechanical disruption of the angle structures and posterior movement of the lens-iris diaphragm, tearing the vessels of the iris and ciliary body and inducing bleeding into the anterior chamber [102]. IOP may then rise and remain elevated until resolution of the hyphema occurs. Even though initial bleeding might be self-limiting due to high IOP, secondary vasospasm of the leaking vessels, and clot formation, with clearing of the hyphema via the fibrinolytic system within the first few days after trauma, open-angle glaucoma may complicate the course of traumatic hyphema when bleeding is relatively long-standing or when rebleeding occurs, secondary to trabecular damage and/or trabecular meshwork obstruction with RBCs, inflammatory cells, and fibrin [103]. Late-onset angle-closure glaucoma can subsequently ensue secondary to fibrosis and posterior and/or peripheral anterior synechiae (PAS) formation.

Hyphema is best quantified at baseline and each follow-up visit at the slit lamp by measuring the height of blood and/or blood clot in the anterior chamber. Hyphema can be red or black, where red is fresh bleeding that can settle and become layered and black is due to deoxygenated, relatively long-standing blood (total black hyphema is called eight-ball hyphema). Rebleeding, seen as an increase in the amount of blood, a layer of red blood or floating RBCs over previously documented clot or darker blood, or, in total hyphema, the new onset of bright red blood at the periphery of the clot, is a common complication, particularly in African-Americans, patients with sickle cell disease or trait, patients on anticoagulant and antiplatelet therapy, patients with bleeding disorders, and those with high IOP and/or low vision at presentation [104, 105]. It can increase the risk of complications including corneal blood staining, high IOP, glaucoma progression, and PAS formation [102].

The degree of IOP elevation in hyphema appears to correlate with the amount of bleeding in the anterior chamber [100], except in sickle cell disease or trait, where minimal bleeding may result in significant IOP elevation [97, 102, 106, 107]. Pressures up to 50 mmHg can be tolerated for 5 days without sustaining damage to the optic nerve (IOP up to 24 mmHg for 24 h in patients with sickle cell disease or trait) [108, 109].

Corneal blood staining occurs almost exclusively in hyphemas larger than one-half anterior chamber height [110, 111]. The cornea should be examined daily at the slit lamp to detect microscopic corneal blood staining in early stages as it initially appears as subtle, small yellowish granules present in the posterior third of the corneal stroma, which may be difficult to recognize against the dark background of blood in the anterior chamber [108]. Another early sign of corneal blood staining when still minimal is biomicroscopic blurriness or loss of sharpness of the ordinarily well-defined fibrillary structure of the posterior corneal stroma on high magnification. These early signs are important to detect, since they usually precede gross corneal blood staining by 24 h, and may warrant surgical intervention to hasten corneal clearing and prevent permanent staining.

Patients with traumatic hyphema should also be evaluated daily to rule out the occurrence of the other above complications and to treat them in a prompt, timely manner when they do occur. Associated ocular injuries (e.g., iridodialysis, lens dislocation/subluxation, or cataract) may become apparent for the first time as the hyphema clears on follow-up visits. Patients should be confined to bed rest or minimal physical activity with head of the bed elevated 30–45° to allow blood to settle and prevent rebleeding. A protective plastic eye shield should be worn at all times. Patching should be avoided as it may delay the patient's recognition of sudden reduction in vision, which is often related to rebleeding. Hospitalization of patients with rebleeding, higher risk of complications such as those with sickle cell disease or trait, patients with associated ocular and/or extraocular injuries, and patients in whom surgical intervention is planned should be considered.

The main goals of initial medical treatment of hyphema are:

- Hastening hyphema clearance
- Prevention of rebleeding
- Management of elevated IOP

Initial medical treatment includes cycloplegic/mydriatic agents, mild analgesics, and topical steroids as described in the Sect. 2.4.9.1. Antifibrinolytic agents such as aminocaproic acid and tranexamic acid can stabilize blood clots in the anterior chamber and prevent rebleeding, with evidence suggesting they significantly reduce the risk of secondary hemorrhage [97, 98, 102, 112]. IOP-lowering therapy as described above is generally initiated when IOP reaches 30 mmHg (24 mmHg in sickle cell disease or trait patients). Nausea and vomiting, if present, may be treated by intramuscular antiemetics (e.g., prochlorperazine) in hospitalized patients, transdermally (e.g., promethazine) or by suppositories in younger children.

Surgical intervention in traumatic hyphema is rarely indicated in hyphemas that occupy less than one-half the anterior chamber [108] and is generally prone to many complications [113]. When indicated, it is aimed at evacuating the anterior chamber blood clots and/or lowering IOP. Evacuating the anterior chamber blood clots is carried out by anterior chamber washout. Indications for this procedure are [97, 98, 114]:

- Four days after onset of total hyphema
- Large persistent hyphema failing to resolve to <50 % anterior chamber height in 8 days
- Significant reduction of visual acuity
- Microscopic corneal blood staining (at any time)
- Uncontrolled IOP >60 mmHg for 2 days
- Uncontrolled IOP >50 mmHg for 5 days

- Uncontrolled IOP >35 mmHg for 7 days
- Uncontrolled IOP >24 mmHg for 24 h in patients with sickle cell disease or trait
- Children at high risk of amblyopia

Surgery should not be delayed in patients with the above indications, since the likelihood of developing gross corneal stromal blood staining and/or glaucomatous optic atrophy is high. Surgical intervention should be preceded by lowering IOP with mannitol and/or systemic carbonic anhydrase inhibitors and is performed in the operating room using the surgical microscope under general anesthesia. Evacuation of hyphema can be done by means of small incision irrigation/aspiration, by evacuation with vitrectomy instrumentation, or, when relatively small, by simple paracentesis [115]. Small incision irrigation/aspiration can be achieved by a single or double needle technique. It carries the risk of injury to the iris and/or lens, possibly inducing iridodialysis when the blood clot in the anterior chamber is large enough to obscure the surgeon's view. It also has the disadvantage of being incomplete, since the fibrinous components are usually left behind.

Evacuation of the blood clots by the vitrectomy instrumentation gives superior results and has the advantage of complete removal of the fibrinous component of the clot. However, it requires a considerable expertise and may not be available in all centers. Simple paracentesis, on the other hand, while may relieve the acutely elevated IOP, may not considerably decrease the volume of the hyphema/blood clots.

In patients with persistent total hyphema and uncontrolled IOP, anterior chamber washout/clot evacuation may be combined with trabeculectomy without antimetabolites (orphan trabeculectomy) with or without peripheral iridectomy. The authors find this technique very useful in this subset of patients, as it serves the purpose of early postoperative lowering of IOP, and thus guarding against the development of glaucomatous optic atrophy, without exposing the patient to the long-term risks of augmented trabeculectomy, since long-term IOP control might not be needed after the resolution of the hyphema. Surgical intervention may also be undertaken to manage long-term complications such as synechiolysis for posterior synechiae or PAS, corneal transplant surgery for permanent, visually significant corneal stromal blood staining, and glaucoma drainage implant (GDI) surgery for patients who develop persistently high IOP and sustain glaucomatous damage despite initial medical and/or surgical therapy. Associated ocular conditions such as traumatic cataract and iridodialysis are also surgically managed at a later stage.

2.4.9.3 Angle Recession Glaucoma

Traumatic angle recession (Fig. 2.17a, b) represents the presence of a tear between the longitudinal and circular fibers of the ciliary muscle. While the term "angle recession glaucoma" may convey the notion that glaucoma in this clinical entity is caused by traumatic angle recession, the term merely indicates that the eye sustained significant trauma that is severe enough to result in retrodisplacement of the iris root and depending of the anterior chamber angle, and while these findings are associated with elevated IOP, they are not the direct causal mechanism of the resultant glaucoma [116]. Angle recession is a common finding after blunt mechanical trauma to the eye, and some degree of angle recession is present in the majority of eyes with traumatic hyphema [117, 118]. However, only 7–9 % of eyes with traumatic angle recession develop glaucoma [119, 120].

Although a larger extent of gonioscopic angle recession (189–240°) has been linked to a higher risk of glaucoma development [91], it is likely that those who develop glaucoma after traumatic angle recession already possess other predisposing factors, and trauma may only be an initiating factor, due to the associated reduced outflow facility secondary to tearing and later scarring of the trabecular meshwork [117, 121]. This is evidenced by the eventual development of glaucoma in the fellow eye in up to 50 % of those who develop glaucoma in association with traumatic angle recession in one eye [122]. Moreover, advanced age is associated with more frequent development of glaucoma in eyes with traumatic angle recession [121].

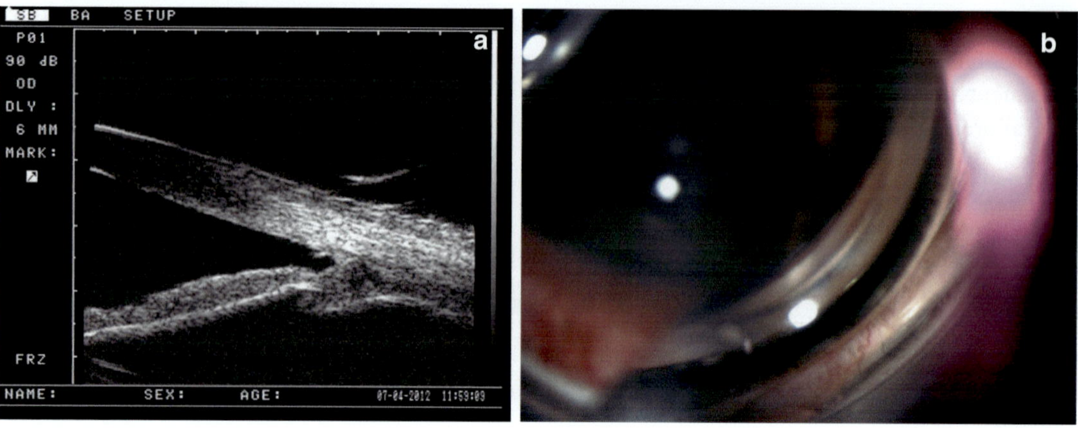

Fig. 2.17 Traumatic angle recession on UBM (**a**) and gonioscope (**b**)

Patients are usually examined in the setting of acute mechanical ocular trauma or may be seen long after trauma. Patients with a relatively remote history of trauma are typically asymptomatic. Slit lamp biomicroscopy may reveal discrepancy between anterior chamber depths in the two eyes. Biomicroscopy may also reveal signs of coincidental iridodialysis, cyclodialysis, iridodonesis, traumatic cataract, Vossius ring (imprinting of iris pigment on the anterior lens surface from forced compression), lens dislocation/subluxation, posterior vitreous detachment (PVD), and retinal dialysis, tears, and/or detachment. IOP may or may not be elevated. Careful gonioscopy, however, remains the only tool to diagnose and confirm traumatic angle recession. Gonioscopic findings include widening of the ciliary body band and abnormal whitening and prominence of the scleral spur. Peripheral anterior synechiae (PAS) may also be observed gonioscopically. Comparison with the other eye is helpful in cases in which angle recession is extensive.

Angle recession glaucoma may take many years to develop. Baseline and annual gonioscopic examination, careful optic nerve head assessment, and IOP measurement should therefore be performed. Baseline Humphrey visual field tests and retinal nerve fiber layer (RNFL) analysis by optical coherence tomography (OCT) may also be performed at baseline and as dictated by clinical suspicion of glaucoma development thereafter.

Surgical closure of the anatomic cleft within the ciliary muscle in traumatic angle recession is usually not attempted. Treatment, whether medical, laser, or surgical, is initiated when IOP rises and glaucoma ensues. IOP-lowering medical treatment is described in the Sect. 2.4.9.1. Selective laser trabeculoplasty (SLT) using Nd:YAG laser is associated with a very high failure rate (up to 100 %) and is generally not recommended by the authors in angle recession glaucoma [123]. Filtration surgery is thought to be less effective in angle recession glaucoma than in primary open-angle glaucoma (POAG), and traumatic angle recession is considered a risk factor for failure of trabeculectomy [124]. However, the use of mitomycin-C (MMC) in trabeculectomy has resulted in better success rates in angle recession glaucoma [125]. Safety and efficacy data of GDI surgery in angle recession glaucoma are scarce, with one study reporting relatively poor outcomes following Molteno tube implantation [126]. Other procedures such as iStent trabecular bypass (Glaukos Corp. Laguna Hills, CA, USA) and diode cyclodestructive procedures have also been used in patients with angle recession glaucoma [127–129].

2.4.9.4 Inflammatory Glaucoma

Intraocular inflammation is a major cause of traumatic glaucoma. It can result in elevation of IOP due to increased inflammatory mediators, cells, and proteins or trabecular meshwork cell dysfunction/trabeculitis, with eventual increased resistance to aqueous outflow [130]. Prolonged or recurrent inflammation may result in posterior and/or peripheral anterior synechiae formation, with secondary pupillary block or angle-closure glaucoma [95]. Inflammatory glaucoma secondary to mechanical ocular trauma may be associated with injuries to various ocular structures, depending on the mechanism and extent of trauma.

Inflammatory glaucomas may be self-limiting or may only require medical treatment as explained in the "General Considerations for the Management of Traumatic Glaucomas" section above. In cases where intraocular inflammation and IOP elevation cannot be adequately controlled with corticosteroid and IOP-lowering therapy, various laser and surgical procedures may be employed. The selection of treatment modality depends on the degree of intraocular inflammation, degree of IOP elevation, angle status, whether posterior and/or peripheral anterior synechiae are present, and the presence of concurrent injury to other ocular structures such as the lens and/or the iris.

Nd:YAG laser peripheral iridotomy (LPI) for pupillary block or angle-closure glaucoma secondary to intraocular inflammation may be ineffective, or even dangerous, given the close proximity of the corneal endothelium to the peripheral iris and the potential for the LPI to close in the setting of continued intraocular inflammation. More than one LPI may therefore be necessary in inflammatory pupillary block, to ensure patency of at least one of them. Surgical peripheral iridectomy with or without posterior and/or anterior peripheral synechiolysis is indicated in cases of LPI failure.

Traditional filtration surgery (i.e., trabeculectomy) as well as non-penetrating surgeries (e.g., deep sclerectomy) and a range of minimally invasive glaucoma surgeries (MIGS) can be employed when IOP is not adequately controlled by the above measures [95]. The authors' primary surgical procedure of choice is Baerveldt glaucoma drainage implant (GDI) placement to achieve efficient, long-lasting control of IOP in inflammatory glaucomas.

2.4.9.5 Trabecular Meshwork Disruption

Glaucoma secondary to trabecular meshwork disruption results from traumatic full- or partial-thickness tears involving the trabecular meshwork [131, 132]. Trabecular disruption may be clinically evident within 48 h of trauma [133]. It can be associated with intraocular inflammation, angle recession, and injury to other ocular structures. Evaluation is best achieved by comparing gonioscopic examination findings in the two eyes. Early gonioscopic findings suggesting trabecular disruption include [89]:

- Partial-thickness flap tears of the trabecular meshwork in the vicinity of the scleral spur
- Full-thickness trabecular meshwork lacerations with exposure of the outer wall of the Schlemm canal
- Sharply demarcated hemorrhage or blood clots in the Schlemm canal
- Torn iris processes
- Excessively prominent scleral spur
- Concomitant angle recession

These changes may obstruct aqueous outflow raise IOP. Mechanical disruption of the trabecular meshwork is usually self-limiting, but pharmacologic treatment using cycloplegic-mydriatic agents, topical corticosteroids, and aqueous suppressants (e.g., β-blockers and CAIs) may often be needed. Constant follow-up is mandated when prompt reduction of IOP is not achieved in a reasonable time for possible intervention as deemed necessary.

2.4.9.6 Phacomorphic Glaucoma

Phacomorphic glaucoma in the setting of mechanical ocular trauma occurs when the crystalline lens fibers are disrupted in an intact capsular bag, causing rapid swelling and enlargement of the anteroposterior diameter of the lens, which may result in pupillary block [134]. Patients may complain of intense ocular pain and nausea due to the rapid elevation of IOP to extreme levels. Clinical examination may reveal:

- Epithelial corneal edema
- Shallowing of the anterior chamber

- Sluggishly reacting, mid-dilated pupil
- Swelling of the crystalline lens with pupillary block
- Dense cataract

Intraocular pressure (IOP) should be medically lowered upon presentation as described in the "General Considerations for the Management of Traumatic Glaucomas" section above. A laser peripheral iridotomy (LPI), although can be effective at relieving the pupillary block, deepening the anterior chamber, and lowering the IOP, is usually difficult to undertake initially due to poor visibility secondary to corneal edema and the proximity of the iris to the corneal endothelium. It can be attempted after initial pharmacologic lowering of the IOP. However, cataract extraction remains the only definitive treatment for phacomorphic glaucoma.

2.4.9.7 Phacoanaphylactic Glaucoma

Phacoanaphylaxis is lens protein-triggered autoimmune reaction that occurs when the capsular bag is disrupted secondary to trauma or surgery (or spontaneously in age-related cataract), exposing the antigenic lens proteins. This immunologic reaction manifests as a granulomatous uveitis occurring after a period of sensitization. The mechanism of IOP elevation and secondary open-angle glaucoma is similar to that in inflammatory glaucoma, where cells and inflammatory debris obstruct the trabecular meshwork and impede aqueous outflow. Definitive diagnosis is made after cataract extraction is performed with histopathologic confirmation of intense inflammatory infiltration of the lens capsule, with the presence of giant cells characteristic of granulomatous inflammation.

Phacoanaphylactic glaucoma may respond to intense topical corticosteroid therapy with or without IOP-lowering treatment. However, similar to all lens-induced glaucomas, the only definitive treatment is cataract extraction. Cataract extraction should not be delayed to minimize sensitization and prevent the development of sympathetic ophthalmia [102], although these recommendations are controversial and no strong evidence supporting them exists.

2.4.9.8 Lens Particle Glaucoma

This type of secondary open-angle glaucoma occurs when the lens capsule is grossly disrupted, allowing lens particles to be released into the anterior chamber and block the aqueous outflow pathway, leading to IOP elevation and secondary glaucoma. Floating or lodged lens particles may induce an intense inflammatory reaction with peripheral and/or anterior peripheral synechia formation, causing pupillary block or secondary angle-closure glaucoma. Medical treatment aimed at reducing intraocular inflammation, preventing or breaking synechiae, and lowering IOP should be promptly initiated. Surgical treatment involving removal of all lens matter and cataract extraction should then be performed to guard against long-term complications.

2.4.9.9 Glaucoma Associated with Lens Subluxation/Dislocation

Lens subluxation/dislocation can occur after sustaining usually a blunt but also possibly a penetrating trauma to the eye. Anterior dislocation may result in pupillary block glaucoma, while posterior dislocation may cause vitreous strands to prolapse through the pupil and also cause a pupillary block glaucoma [102]. Synechial formation may develop in neglected cases, and chronic synechial angle closure may ensue. Medical management of glaucoma associated with lens subluxation/dislocation should be given as necessary. However, early definitive treatment as described in the Sect. 2.4.8 should be done on an urgent basis to prevent the potentially harmful complications associated with lens subluxation/dislocation. Multiple laser peripheral iridotomies (LPIs) may be done while awaiting surgical correction, since the unstable lens may move and occlude the iridotomy if only one is performed [103].

2.4.9.10 Ghost Cell Glaucoma

Ghost cell glaucoma is caused by degenerated, senescent red blood cells blocking the trabecular meshwork in the setting of vitreous hemorrhage and disrupted anterior vitreous face [135]. However, it can also occur with long-standing hyphema in the absence of vitreous hemorrhage [102]. Its onset is usually 2–3 weeks following the inciting trauma [135]. The degree of IOP elevation correlates with the number of ghost cells in the anterior chamber [103].

Ghost cell glaucoma is characterized by pain and corneal edema. Slit lamp examination reveals characteristic khaki-colored cells floating in the anterior chamber and deposited on the endothelium and anterior vitreous face. Pseudohypopyon may be present, and mixing of ghost cells with layers of fresh blood may give the characteristic "candy stripe" appearance. Diagnosis is confirmed by demonstration of hollow, thin-walled erythrocytes with clumps of denatured hemoglobin (Heinz bodies) in an aqueous aspirate specimen [136].

Initial treatment involves pharmacologic IOP-lowering therapy. However, pharmacologic therapy may not be sufficient in many cases in which dense hemorrhage is present or IOP is not adequately controlled [135]. Surgical intervention to allow complete removal of ghost cells by anterior chamber washout and/or vitrectomy is indicated in these cases.

2.4.9.11 Hemolytic Glaucoma

When mechanical ocular trauma results in intraocular hemorrhage, hemoglobin-laden macrophages, free hemoglobin, and lysed erythrocyte remnants may block the trabecular meshwork several days to weeks after the onset of hemorrhage, posing resistance to aqueous outflow and raising IOP [137]. A secondary open-angle glaucoma may then ensue if long-standing or when the volume of hemolytic debris is relatively large. Diagnosis is largely clinical, and slit lamp examination may reveal reddish brown small cells in the anterior chamber on high magnification. Gonioscopic examination often shows reddish brown trabecular meshwork and an open angle. Confirmation by cytological examination of an aqueous aspirate specimen to demonstrate hemoglobin-laden macrophages may sometimes be indicated to rule out malignancy [138].

Hemolytic glaucoma is usually self-limiting, and pharmacologic IOP-lowering therapy is the first-line treatment of choice. However, anterior chamber washout and/or vitrectomy to eliminate the source of bleeding is indicated in recalcitrant cases.

2.4.9.12 Hemosiderotic Glaucoma

Hemosiderotic glaucoma is a rare secondary open-angle glaucoma that is seen after long-standing intraocular hemorrhage [139]. In prolonged intraocular bleeding, trabecular meshwork endothelial cells absorb iron, which is a product of hemoglobin degradation from lysed erythrocytes. When the apoferritin-ferritin intracellular iron-storage mechanism becomes saturates, toxic inorganic iron granules accumulate within the trabecular meshwork endothelial cells, resulting in siderosis and obstruction of intertrabecular spaces, which may impede aqueous outflow and raise IOP.

Initial management of hemosiderotic glaucoma involves pharmacologic lowering of IOP, as explained in the "General Considerations for the Management of Traumatic Glaucomas" section above. However, filtration surgery or glaucoma drainage implant surgery is indicated when advanced siderotic angle damage is present. Anterior chamber washout and/or vitrectomy may also be required to eliminate the source of intraocular hemorrhage.

Acknowledgement The authors thank the colleagues of Dr. Hua Yan who provided all of the Figures for this book chapter.

Clinical pearls in the management of anterior segment trauma

- Thorough history taking is important in guiding further assessment, diagnostic testing, and treatment modalities employed in the management of mechanical ocular trauma.
- Placement of a protective eye shield rather than an eye patch is strongly recommended when ocular examination is not being carried out when an open globe injury is suspected.
- Undue strain (e.g., placing a lid speculum or assessing ocular motility) should be avoided on a suspected open globe.
- Differentiating traumatic mydriasis from pre-existing mydriasis is important.

- Conservative pharmacologic treatment of traumatic mydriasis with competitive α-adrenergic antagonists should be attempted before surgical correction is planned.
- Early, prompt surgical management of prolapsed iris tissue not adequately covered by conjunctiva is of paramount importance to avoid iridocorneal adhesions, endophthalmitis, surface epithelialization and epithelial down growth, and secondary angle closure glaucoma.
- Small iridodialyses or those adequately covered by the upper eyelid are usually asymptomatic and may be observed.
- Opaque, iris-print contact lenses may be used in traumatic aniridia when lens surgery is not planned.
- Leak from an occult open globe wound should be ruled out before the diagnosis of traumatic hypotony is considered.
- Minimally leaking or self-sealing wounds can be managed conservatively with pressure patching or bandage contact lens placement and topical aqueous suppressants.
- Ultrasound biomicroscopy (UBM) and anterior segment optical coherence tomography (AS-OCT) are commonly used in the diagnosis and evaluation of cyclodialysis clefts.
- The timing of surgery to correct traumatic lens surgery is controversial. Primary surgery is recommended for faster visual rehabilitation, reduced inflammation, avoiding lens-induced IOP rise and refractive fluctuations, and relieving vitreoretinal traction. Delayed surgery is recommended in small, visually insignificant cataracts, and when resources and/or specialized surgical expertise not available at the time of primary surgery are needed.
- Medical therapy alone is usually not sufficient to control traumatic glaucoma, and complex surgical procedures to restore normal ocular anatomy, address coexisting traumatic ocular injuries, and/or lower IOP are often necessary.
- Topical and systemic CAIs and hyperosmotic agents should be avoided in patients with sickle cell disease or trait.
- Patients with traumatic hyphema should be evaluated daily at the slitlamp, and a protective plastic eye shield should be worn at all times.
- Hospitalization of traumatic hyphema patients with rebleeding, higher risk of complications (e.g., sickle cell disease or trait), and patients with associated ocular injuries, should be considered.
- Initial medical treatment of traumatic hyphema includes cycloplegic/mydriatic agents, mild analgesics, topical steroids, and, IOP-lowering therapy.
- Prompt surgical intervention in traumatic hyphema by means of anterior chamber washout/clot evacuation with or without unaugmented trabeculectomy is indicated when there is significant reduction of visual acuity, corneal blood staining, medically uncontrolled IOP, or in children prone to amblyopia.
- Baseline and annual gonioscopic examination, careful optic nerve head assessment and IOP measurement should be performed for early detection of late-onset angle recession glaucoma.
- More than one LPI may be necessary in inflammatory pupillary block to ensure patency of at least one LPI.
- Laser peripheral iridotomy (LPI is usually difficult to undertake initially in cases of phacomorphic glaucoma, and cataract extraction remains the only definitive treatment.
- Phacoanaphylactic glaucoma may respond to intense topical corticosteroid therapy with or without IOP-lowering treatment, with cataract extraction being the only definitive treatment.
- Surgical intervention by anterior chamber washout and/or vitrectomy is indicated in ghost cell glaucoma when initial medical therapy fails to control IOP and/or resolve dense hemorrhage.

References

1. Mukherjee P, Sivakumar A. Tetanus prophylaxis in superficial corneal abrasions. Emerg Med J. 2003;20(1):62–4.
2. Boldt HC, Pulido JS, Blodi CF, et al. Rural endophthalmitis. Ophthalmology. 1989;96(12):1722–6.
3. Bai HQ, Yao L, Wang DB, et al. Causes and treatments of traumatic secondary glaucoma. Eur J Ophthalmol. 2009;19(2):201–6.
4. Sharma A, Votruba M. Thymoxamine in the treatment of traumatic mydriasis. Br J Ophthalmol. 1993; 77(10):681.
5. Ogawa GS. The iris cerclage suture for permanent mydriasis: a running suture technique. Ophthalmic Surg Lasers. 1998;29(12):1001–9.
6. Siepser SB. The closed chamber slipping suture technique for iris repair. Ann Ophthalmol. 1994;26(3):71–2.
7. Barlow A, Weiner HL. Traumatic iridodialysis; its surgical correction. Arch Ophthal. 1945;34:292–4.
8. McCannel MA. A retrievable suture idea for anterior uveal problems. Ophthalmic Surg. 1976;7(2):98–103.
9. Wachler BB, Krueger RR. Double-armed McCannell suture for repair of traumatic iridodialysis. Am J Ophthalmol. 1996;122(1):109–10.
10. Romem M, Singer L. Traumatic aniridia. Br J Ophthalmol. 1973;57(8):613–4.
11. Qiu X, Ji Y, Zheng T, Lu Y. Long-term efficacy and complications of black diaphragm intraocular lens implantation in patients with traumatic aniridia. Br J Ophthalmol. 2015;99(5):659–64.
12. Srinivasan S, Ting DS, Snyder ME, et al. Prosthetic iris devices. Can J Ophthalmol. 2014;49(1):6–17.
13. Costa VP, Arcieri ES. Hypotony maculopathy. Acta Ophthalmol Scand. 2007;85(6):586–97.
14. Pederson JE. Ocular hypotony. Trans Ophthalmol Soc U K. 1986;105(Pt 2):220–6.
15. Aminlari A, Callahan CE. Medical, laser, and surgical management of inadvertent cyclodialysis cleft with hypotony. Arch Ophthalmol. 2004;122(3):399–404.
16. Razeghinejad MR, Dehghani C. Effect of ocular hypotony secondary to cyclodialysis cleft on corneal topography. Cornea. 2008;27(5):609–11.
17. Ding C, Zeng J. Clinical study on hypotony following blunt ocular trauma. Int J Ophthalmol. 2012;5(6):771–3.
18. Kucukerdonmez C, Beutel J, Bartz-Schmidt KU, Gelisken F. Treatment of chronic ocular hypotony with intraocular application of sodium hyaluronate. Br J Ophthalmol. 2009;93(2):235–9.
19. Kuhl D, Mieler W. Ciliary body. In: Kuhn F, Pieramici D, editors. Ocular trauma principles and practice. New York: Thieme New York; 2002.
20. Yang JG, Yao GM, Li SP, et al. Surgical treatment for 42 patients with traumatic annular ciliochoroidal detachment. Int J Ophthalmol. 2011;4(1):81–4.
21. Ormerod LD, Baerveldt G, Sunalp MA, Riekhof FT. Management of the hypotonous cyclodialysis cleft. Ophthalmology. 1991;98(9):1384–93.
22. Suguro K, Toris CB, Pederson JE. Uveoscleral outflow following cyclodialysis in the monkey eye using a fluorescent tracer. Invest Ophthalmol Vis Sci. 1985;26(6):810–3.
23. Kronfeld PC. The fluid exchange in the successfully cyclodialyzed eye. Trans Am Ophthalmol Soc. 1954;52:249–63.
24. Shaffer RN, Weiss DI. Concerning cyclodialysis and hypotony. Arch Ophthalmol. 1962;68:25–31.
25. Ioannidis AS, Barton K. Cyclodialysis cleft: causes and repair. Curr Opin Ophthalmol. 2010;21(2):150–4.
26. Joondeph HC. Management of postoperative and post-traumatic cyclodialysis clefts with argon laser photocoagulation. Ophthalmic Surg. 1980;11(3):186–8.
27. Harbin Jr TS. Treatment of cyclodialysis clefts with argon laser photocoagulation. Ophthalmology. 1982;89(9):1082–3.
28. Amini H, Razeghinejad MR. Transscleral diode laser therapy for cyclodialysis cleft induced hypotony. Clin Experiment Ophthalmol. 2005;33(4):348–50.
29. Brown SV, Mizen T. Transscleral diode laser therapy for traumatic cyclodialysis cleft. Ophthalmic Surg Lasers. 1997;28(4):313–7.
30. Barasch K, Galin MA, Baras I. Postcyclodialysis hypotony. Am J Ophthalmol. 1969;68(4):644–5.
31. Maumenee AE, Stark WJ. Management of persistent hypotony after planned or inadvertent cyclodialysis. Am J Ophthalmol. 1971;71(1 Pt 2):320–7.
32. Krohn J. Cryotherapy in the treatment of cyclodialysis cleft induced hypotony. Acta Ophthalmol Scand. 1997;75(1):96–8.
33. Ceruti P, Tosi R, Marchini G. Gas tamponade and cyclocryotherapy of a chronic cyclodialysis cleft. Br J Ophthalmol. 2009;93(3):414–6.
34. Spiegel D, Katz LJ, McNamara JA. Surgical repair of a traumatic cyclodialysis cleft after laser failure. Ophthalmic Surg. 1990;21(5):372–3.
35. Lamkin JC, Azar DT, Mead MD, Volpe NJ. Simultaneous corneal laceration repair, cataract removal, and posterior chamber intraocular lens implantation. Am J Ophthalmol. 1992;113(6):626–31.
36. Berinstein DM, Gentile RC, Sidoti PA, et al. Ultrasound biomicroscopy in anterior ocular trauma. Ophthalmic Surg Lasers. 1997;28(3):201–7.
37. Boorstein JM, Titelbaum DS, Patel Y, et al. CT diagnosis of unsuspected traumatic cataracts in patients with complicated eye injuries: significance of attenuation value of the lens. AJR Am J Roentgenol. 1995;164(1):181–4.
38. Grewal SP, Jain R, Gupta R, Grewal D. Role of scheimpflug imaging in traumatic intralenticular foreign body. Am J Ophthalmol. 2006;142(4):675–6.
39. Singh R, Ram J, Gupta R. Use of Scheimpflug imaging in the management of intra-lenticular foreign body. Nepal J Ophthalmol. 2015;7(13):82–4.
40. McElvanney AM, Talbot EM. Posterior chamber lens implantation combined with pars plana vitrectomy. J Cataract Refract Surg. 1997;23(1):106–10.
41. Almog Y, Reider-Groswasser I, Goldstein M, et al. "The disappearing lens": failure of CT to image the

lens in traumatic intumescent cataract. J Comput Assist Tomogr. 1999;23(3):354–6.
42. Keeney AH. Intralenticular foreign bodies. Arch Ophthalmol. 1971;86(5):499–501.
43. Klemen UM, Freyler H. Siderosis bulbi et lentis produced by intralenticular rust (author's transl). Klin Monbl Augenheilkd. 1978;172(2):258–61.
44. Mester V, Kuhn F. Lens. In: Kuhn F, Pieramici D, editors. Ocular trauma principles and practice. New York: Thieme New York; 2002.
45. Osher RH. Slow motion phacoemulsification approach. J Cataract Refract Surg. 1993;19(5):667.
46. Lifshitz T, Levy J, Kratz A, et al. Planned posterior assisted levitation in severe subluxated cataract: surgical technique and clinical results. Indian J Ophthalmol. 2012;60(6):567–9.
47. Eckstein M, Vijayalakshmi P, Killedar M, et al. Use of intraocular lenses in children with traumatic cataract in south India. Br J Ophthalmol. 1998;82(8):911–5.
48. Malukiewicz-Wisniewska G, Kaluzny J, Lesiewska-Junk H, Eliks I. Intraocular lens implantation in children and youth. J Pediatr Ophthalmol Strabismus. 1999;36(3):129–33.
49. Nihalani BR, VanderVeen DK. Technological advances in pediatric cataract surgery. Semin Ophthalmol. 2010;25(5–6):271–4.
50. Hazirolan DO, Altiparmak UE, Aslan BS, Duman S. Vitrectorhexis versus forceps capsulorhexis for anterior and posterior capsulotomy in congenital cataract surgery. J Pediatr Ophthalmol Strabismus. 2009;46(2):104–7.
51. Kochgaway L, Biswas P, Paul A, et al. Vitrectorhexis versus forceps posterior capsulorhexis in pediatric cataract surgery. Indian J Ophthalmol. 2013;61(7):361–4.
52. Assia EI, Legler UF, Apple DJ. The capsular bag after short- and long-term fixation of intraocular lenses. Ophthalmology. 1995;102(8):1151–7.
53. Chang DF. Single versus three piece acrylic IOLs. Br J Ophthalmol. 2004;88(6):727–8.
54. Davison JA. Capsule contraction syndrome. J Cataract Refract Surg. 1993;19(5):582–9.
55. Hayashi H, Hayashi K, Nakao F, Hayashi F. Anterior capsule contraction and intraocular lens dislocation in eyes with pseudoexfoliation syndrome. Br J Ophthalmol. 1998;82(12):1429–32.
56. Rubsamen PE, Irvin WD, McCuen 2nd BW, et al. Primary intraocular lens implantation in the setting of penetrating ocular trauma. Ophthalmology. 1995;102(1):101–7.
57. Holt DG, Young J, Stagg B, Ambati BK. Anterior chamber intraocular lens, sutured posterior chamber intraocular lens, or glued intraocular lens: where do we stand? Curr Opin Ophthalmol. 2012;23(1):62–7.
58. Sawada T, Kimura W, Kimura T, et al. Long-term follow-up of primary anterior chamber intraocular lens implantation. J Cataract Refract Surg. 1998;24(11):1515–20.
59. Smith PW, Wong SK, Stark WJ, et al. Complications of semiflexible, closed-loop anterior chamber intraocular lenses. Arch Ophthalmol. 1987;105(1):52–7.
60. Li J, Yuan G, Ying L, et al. Modified implantation of black diaphragm intraocular lens in traumatic aniridia. J Cataract Refract Surg. 2013;39(6):822–5.
61. Maggi R, Maggi C. Sutureless scleral fixation of intraocular lenses. J Cataract Refract Surg. 1997;23(9):1289–94.
62. Gabor SG, Pavlidis MM. Sutureless intrascleral posterior chamber intraocular lens fixation. J Cataract Refract Surg. 2007;33(11):1851–4.
63. Scharioth GB, Prasad S, Georgalas I, et al. Intermediate results of sutureless intrascleral posterior chamber intraocular lens fixation. J Cataract Refract Surg. 2010;36(2):254–9.
64. Ganekal S, Venkataratnam S, Dorairaj S, Jhanji V. Comparative evaluation of suture-assisted and fibrin glue-assisted scleral fixated intraocular lens implantation. J Refract Surg. 2012;28(4):249–52.
65. Kumar DA, Agarwal A, Agarwal A, et al. Long-term assessment of tilt of glued intraocular lenses: an optical coherence tomography analysis 5 years after surgery. Ophthalmology. 2015;122(1):48–55.
66. Agarwal A, Kumar DA, Jacob S, et al. Fibrin glue-assisted sutureless posterior chamber intraocular lens implantation in eyes with deficient posterior capsules. J Cataract Refract Surg. 2008;34(9):1433–8.
67. Kumar DA, Agarwal A, Jacob S, et al. Combined surgical management of capsular and iris deficiency with glued intraocular lens technique. J Refract Surg. 2013;29(5):342–7.
68. Ahmedbegovic Pjano M, Alikadic-Husovic A, Grisevic S, et al. Efficacy and safety of iris-supported phakic lenses (Verisyse) for treating moderately high myopia. Med Glas (Zenica). 2016;13(1):25.
69. Bouheraoua N, Bonnet C, Labbe A, et al. Iris-fixated phakic intraocular lens implantation to correct myopia and a predictive model of endothelial cell loss. J Cataract Refract Surg. 2015;41(11):2450–7.
70. Karimian F, Baradaran-Rafii A, Hashemian SJ, et al. Comparison of three phakic intraocular lenses for correction of myopia. J Ophthalmic Vis Res. 2014;9(4):427–33.
71. Guell JL, Verdaguer P, Elies D, et al. Secondary iris-claw anterior chamber lens implantation in patients with aphakia without capsular support. Br J Ophthalmol. 2014;98(5):658–63.
72. Teng H, Zhang H, Tian F, et al. Artisan iris claw intraocular lens implantation for the correction of aphakia after pars plana vitrectomy. Zhonghua Yan Ke Za Zhi. 2014;50(2):89–94.
73. Gawdat GI, Taher SG, Salama MM, Ali AA. Evaluation of Artisan aphakic intraocular lens in cases of pediatric aphakia with insufficient capsular support. J AAPOS. 2015;19(3):242–6.
74. Chen Y, Liu Q, Xue C, et al. Three-year follow-up of secondary anterior iris fixation of an aphakic intraocular lens to correct aphakia. J Cataract Refract Surg. 2012;38(9):1595–601.
75. Gonnermann J, Amiri S, Klamann M, et al. Endothelial cell loss after retropupillary iris-claw

intraocular lens implantation. Klin Monbl Augenheilkd. 2014;231(8):784–7.
76. Forlini M, Soliman W, Bratu A, et al. Long-term follow-up of retropupillary iris-claw intraocular lens implantation: a retrospective analysis. BMC Ophthalmol. 2015;15:143.
77. Gonnermann J, Torun N, Klamann MK, et al. Posterior iris-claw aphakic intraocular lens implantation in children. Am J Ophthalmol. 2013;156(2):382–6. e1.
78. Hirashima DE, Soriano ES, Meirelles RL, et al. Outcomes of iris-claw anterior chamber versus iris-fixated foldable intraocular lens in subluxated lens secondary to Marfan syndrome. Ophthalmology. 2010;117(8):1479–85.
79. Por YM, Lavin MJ. Techniques of intraocular lens suspension in the absence of capsular/zonular support. Surv Ophthalmol. 2005;50(5):429–62.
80. Bowman RJ, Yorston D, Wood M, et al. Primary intraocular lens implantation for penetrating lens trauma in Africa. Ophthalmology. 1998;105(9):1770–4.
81. Pavlovic S. Primary intraocular lens implantation during pars plana vitrectomy and intraretinal foreign body removal. Retina. 1999;19(5):430–6.
82. Thouvenin D, Lesueur L, Arne JL. Intercapsular implantation in the management of cataract in children. Study of 87 cases and comparison to 88 cases without implantation. J Fr Ophtalmol. 1995;18(11):678–87.
83. Koenig SB, Ruttum MS, Lewandowski MF, Schultz RO. Pseudophakia for traumatic cataracts in children. Ophthalmology. 1993;100(8):1218–24.
84. Chan TK, Mackintosh G, Yeoh R, Lim AS. Primary posterior chamber IOL implantation in penetrating ocular trauma. Int Ophthalmol. 1993;17(3):137–41.
85. Tyagi AK, Kheterpal S, Callear AB, et al. Simultaneous posterior chamber intraocular lens implant combined with vitreoretinal surgery for intraocular foreign body injuries. Eye (Lond). 1998;12(Pt 2):230–3.
86. Kora Y, Shimizu K, Inatomi M, et al. Eye growth after cataract extraction and intraocular lens implantation in children. Ophthalmic Surg. 1993;24(7):467–75.
87. BenEzra D, Cohen E, Rose L. Traumatic cataract in children: correction of aphakia by contact lens or intraocular lens. Am J Ophthalmol. 1997;123(6):773–82.
88. Lesueur L, Thouvenin D, Arne JL. Visual and sensory results of surgical treatment of cataract in children. Apropos of 135 cases. J Fr Ophtalmol. 1995;18(11):667–77.
89. De Leon-Ortega JE, Girkin CA. Ocular trauma-related glaucoma. Ophthalmol Clin North Am. 2002;15(2):215–23.
90. Girkin CA, McGwin Jr G, Morris R, Kuhn F. Glaucoma following penetrating ocular trauma: a cohort study of the United States Eye Injury Registry. Am J Ophthalmol. 2005;139(1):100–5.
91. Sihota R, Sood NN, Agarwal HC. Traumatic glaucoma. Acta Ophthalmol Scand. 1995;73(3):252–4.
92. May DR, Kuhn FP, Morris RE, et al. The epidemiology of serious eye injuries from the United States Eye Injury Registry. Graefes Arch Clin Exp Ophthalmol. 2000;238(2):153–7.
93. Klopfer J, Tielsch JM, Vitale S, et al. Ocular trauma in the United States. Eye injuries resulting in hospitalization, 1984 through 1987. Arch Ophthalmol. 1992;110(6):838–42.
94. Haring RS, Canner JK, Haider AH, Schneider EB. Ocular injury in the United States: emergency department visits from 2006–2011. Injury. 2016;47:104–8.
95. Sayed MS, Lee RK. Current management approaches for uveitic glaucoma. Int Ophthalmol Clin. 2015;55(3):141–60.
96. Bleiman BS, Schwartz AL. Paradoxical intraocular pressure response to pilocarpine. A proposed mechanism and treatment. Arch Ophthalmol. 1979;97(7):1305–6.
97. Walton W, Von Hagen S, Grigorian R, Zarbin M. Management of traumatic hyphema. Surv Ophthalmol. 2002;47(4):297–334.
98. Sankar PS, Chen TC, Grosskreutz CL, Pasquale LR. Traumatic hyphema. Int Ophthalmol Clin. 2002;42(3):57–68.
99. Romano PE, Robinson JA. Traumatic hyphema: a comprehensive review of the past half century yields 8076 cases for which specific medical treatment reduces rebleeding 62%, from 13% to 5% (P<.0001). Binocul Vis Strabismus Q. 2000;15(2):175–86.
100. Crouch Jr ER, Crouch ER. Management of traumatic hyphema: therapeutic options. J Pediatr Ophthalmol Strabismus. 1999;36(5):238–50; quiz 79–80.
101. ER Crouch J, Williams P. Trauma: ruptures and bleeding. In: Tasman JE, editor. Duane's clinical ophthalmology. Philadelphia: Lippincott; 1993; v. IV.
102. Nuyen B, Mansouri K, Shaarawy TM. Post-traumatic glaucoma. In: Shaarawy TM, Sherwood MB, Hitchings RA, Crowston JG, editors. Glaucoma. 2nd ed. St. Louis: Elsevier Saunders Limited; 2015; v. I.
103. Matelis KH, Congdon N. Glaucoma. In: Kuhn F, Pieramici DJ, editors. Ocular trauma principles and practice. New York: Thieme Medical Publishers, Inc.; 2002.
104. Rahmani B, Jahadi HR, Rajaeefard A. An analysis of risk for secondary hemorrhage in traumatic hyphema. Ophthalmology. 1999;106(2):380–5.
105. Nasrullah A, Kerr NC. Sickle cell trait as a risk factor for secondary hemorrhage in children with traumatic hyphema. Am J Ophthalmol. 1997;123(6):783–90.
106. Lai JC, Fekrat S, Barron Y, Goldberg MF. Traumatic hyphema in children: risk factors for complications. Arch Ophthalmol. 2001;119(1):64–70.
107. Mowatt L, Chambers C. Ocular morbidity of traumatic hyphema in a Jamaican hospital. Eur J Ophthalmol. 2010;20(3):584–9.
108. Read JE, Goldberg MF. Blunt ocular trauma and hyphema. Int Ophthalmol Clin. 1974;14(4):57–97.
109. Cohen SB, Fletcher ME, Goldberg MF, Jednock NJ. Diagnosis and management of ocular complications of sickle hemoglobinopathies: part V. Ophthalmic Surg. 1986;17(6):369–74.

110. Crouch Jr ER, Frenkel M. Aminocaproic acid in the treatment of traumatic hyphema. Am J Ophthalmol. 1976;81(3):355–60.
111. Read J. Traumatic hyphema: surgical vs medical management. Ann Ophthalmol. 1975;7(5):659–62, 64–6, 68–70.
112. Aylward GW, Dunlop IS, Little BC. Meta-analysis of systemic anti-fibrinolytics in traumatic hyphaema. Eye (Lond). 1994;8(Pt 4):440–2.
113. Kutner B, Fourman S, Brein K, et al. Aminocaproic acid reduces the risk of secondary hemorrhage in patients with traumatic hyphema. Arch Ophthalmol. 1987;105(2):206–8.
114. Brandt MT, Haug RH. Traumatic hyphema: a comprehensive review. J Oral Maxillofac Surg. 2001;59(12):1462–70.
115. Nash DL, Sheppard JD. Hyphema. In: Talavera F, Rapuano CJ, editors. eMedicine. Medscape; 2015; v. 2015. Available from: http://emedicine.medscape.com/article/1190165-overview
116. Wolff SM, Zimmerman LE. Chronic secondary glaucoma. Associated with retrodisplacement of iris root and deepening of the anterior chamber angle secondary to contusion. Am J Ophthalmol. 1962; 54:547–63.
117. Blanton FM. Anterior chamber angle recession and secondary glaucoma. A study of the aftereffects of traumatic hyphemas. Arch Ophthalmol. 1964;72:39–43.
118. Canavan YM, Archer DB. Anterior segment consequences of blunt ocular injury. Br J Ophthalmol. 1982;66(9):549–55.
119. Kaufman JH, Tolpin DW. Glaucoma after traumatic angle recession. A ten-year prospective study. Am J Ophthalmol. 1974;78(4):648–54.
120. Mooney D. Angle recession and secondary glaucoma. Br J Ophthalmol. 1973;57(8):608–12.
121. Thiel HJ, Aden G, Pulhorn G. Changes in the chamber angle following ocular contusions (author's transl). Klin Monbl Augenheilkd. 1980;177(2):165–73.
122. Tesluk GC, Spaeth GL. The occurrence of primary open-angle glaucoma in the fellow eye of patients with unilateral angle-cleavage glaucoma. Ophthalmology. 1985;92(7):904–11.
123. Fukuchi T, Iwata K, Sawaguchi S, et al. Nd:YAG laser trabeculopuncture (YLT) for glaucoma with traumatic angle recession. Graefes Arch Clin Exp Ophthalmol. 1993;231(10):571–6.
124. Mermoud A, Salmon JF, Straker C, Murray AD. Post-traumatic angle recession glaucoma: a risk factor for bleb failure after trabeculectomy. Br J Ophthalmol. 1993;77(10):631–4.
125. Manners T, Salmon JF, Barron A, et al. Trabeculectomy with mitomycin C in the treatment of post-traumatic angle recession glaucoma. Br J Ophthalmol. 2001;85(2):159–63.
126. Mermoud A, Salmon JF, Barron A, et al. Surgical management of post-traumatic angle recession glaucoma. Ophthalmology. 1993;100(5):634–42.
127. Schlote T, Derse M, Rassmann K, et al. Efficacy and safety of contact transscleral diode laser cyclophotocoagulation for advanced glaucoma. J Glaucoma. 2001;10(4):294–301.
128. Kivela T, Puska P, Raitta C, et al. Clinically successful contact transscleral krypton laser cyclophotocoagulation. Long-term histopathologic and immunohistochemical autopsy findings. Arch Ophthalmol. 1995;113(11):1447–53.
129. de Klerk TA, Au L. I-Stent for treatment of angle recession with raised intraocular pressure. Clin Experiment Ophthalmol. 2012;40(5):527–8.
130. Kok H, Barton K. Uveitic glaucoma. Ophthalmol Clin North Am. 2002;15(3):375–87, viii.
131. Endo S, Ishida N, Yamaguchi T. Tear in the trabecular meshwork caused by an airsoft gun. Am J Ophthalmol. 2001;131(5):656–7.
132. Herschler J. Trabecular damage due to blunt anterior segment injury and its relationship to traumatic glaucoma. Trans Sect Ophthalmol Am Acad Ophthalmol Otolaryngol. 1977;83(2):239–48.
133. Alper MG. Contusion angle deformity and glaucoma. Gonioscopic observations and clinical course. Arch Ophthalmol. 1963;69:455–67.
134. Epstein DL. Diagnosis and management of lens-induced glaucoma. Ophthalmology. 1982; 89(3):227–30.
135. Campbell DG. Ghost cell glaucoma following trauma. Ophthalmology. 1981;88(11):1151–8.
136. Cameron JD, Havener VR. Histologic confirmation of ghost cell glaucoma by routine light microscopy. Am J Ophthalmol. 1983;96(2):251–2.
137. Fenton RH, Hunter WS. Hemolytic glaucoma. Surv Ophthalmol. 1965;10(4):355–60.
138. Phelps CD, Watzke RC. Hemolytic glaucoma. Am J Ophthalmol. 1975;80(4):690–5.
139. Vannas S. Hemosiderosis in eyes with secondary glaucoma after delayed intraocular hemorrhages. Acta Ophthalmol (Copenh). 1960;38: 254–67.

3 Posterior Segment Trauma

William E. Smiddy

3.1 Introduction

Mechanical ocular trauma involving the posterior segment may result in damage to the choroid, vitreous body, retina, macular and optic nerve, leading to permanent visual impairment or severe visual loss. Complicated cases such as traumatic choroidal hemorrhage, retinal detachment, traumatic macula hole, retinal detachments, and intraocular foreign bodies often bring great challenges to clinicians. Vitreoretinal surgery is usually required in the acute and secondary management of the posterior ocular trauma.

The advent of vitrectomy was over 40 years ago, and while the pace of its development during the first 20 years was extremely rapid with recognition of widening clinical applications, the advances of the past 10 years have centered mostly on small incision surgery techniques and instrumentation to support those efforts [1]. While these developments have generally decreased operating times, the principal application advantages pertain to non-trauma cases. Still, the sorts of considerations in an eye that has sustained trauma have borrowed liberally from techniques and principles from more elective sorts of cases, so this has not been a trivial factor, but it has not been transformative either. Rather, it is the extent of the initial injury and the biological constraints that still limit prognosis in trauma. Hence, the principles that governed the management of trauma 20 years ago are similar to those today: timing and contending with proliferative vitreoretinopathy.

This chapter will offer a review of the principles involved in managing the spectrum of ocular trauma – penetrating trauma, blunt trauma, macular holes, and choroidal hemorrhage – with some attention also to anterior segment conditions that impact the posterior segment such as traumatic lens dislocation.

3.2 Purpose of Intervention

The first step in effectively managing any condition is to establish the objectives of the intervention. For posterior segment trauma, these objectives typically involve reestablishing ocular integrity, clearing media opacities, treating complications such as retinal detachment and proliferations, and taking preemptive measures to prevent retinal detachment. Secondary objectives may become primary objectives for secondary procedures and include contending with lens complications and anterior segment injuries. Injuries limited to the anterior segment, glaucoma, endophthalmitis, and intraocular foreign bodies, as well as features unique to the pediatric population, will be addressed in separate chapters.

W.E. Smiddy, MD, PhD
Department of Ophthalmology, University of Miami Miller School of Medicine, Miami, FL, USA
e-mail: wsmiddy@med.miami.edu

H. Yan (ed.), *Mechanical Ocular Trauma*, DOI 10.1007/978-981-10-2150-3_3

3.3 Prognosis of Eyes After Trauma

Seminal experimental and clinical studies from the 1980s remain important today when assessing and explaining to patients and their families the prognosis [2–9]. More so than in elective cases, primary treatment of trauma is confronted during a time of great turmoil, and the patient is in a vulnerable position due to the sudden tragedy. Moreover, the caregivers, recognizing the severity of the situation, are focused on the immediacy of stabilizing the eye when time and prognostic information is lacking. The ophthalmologist might recognize that the battle is commonly for ambulatory vision, while the patient's expectations commonly are much higher, which is natural since this is a unique situation for them.

The prognosis for even ambulatory vision is poor when there is visual acuity worse than 5/200, an afferent pupillary defect, a corneoscleral defect of >12 mm, and a blunt nature of injury [8–10]. These clinical findings are consistent with the animal model anatomic findings.

3.4 Timing of Intervention

This is probably the most controversial of all of these "hot topics." There is no debate that prompt closure of an open globe should be undertaken as promptly as is reasonably possible, usually within hours, for optimal management. The debate on timing is whether posterior segment objectives should be addressed concurrently or even within 3 days or so of a primary repair, versus waiting a week or so for a secondary repair. The former is unquestionably the choice when there is infection or an intraocular foreign body. However, in the more common circumstance, this is not clear. There is consensus that secondary repair should not be delayed longer than about a week, since thereafter the proliferative process has ramped up in a way that causes irreparable ocular injury. Eyes with vitreous hemorrhage (VH) after a penetrating injury in particular should not be watched conservatively as eyes with a spontaneous VH might be.

Proponents of early vitrectomy present good results and argue that more freshly injured tissues are more pliable and conducive to repair [11]. Furthermore, there is a risk of sympathetic ophthalmia after vitrectomy for trauma, but as rare as that is within 2 weeks of injury, the earliest report is 5 days after surgery [12, 13]; theoretically anatomic repair might lessen this risk and earlier repair might further lower the risk, but this is conjecture. It is this author's bias, as has been advocated by others [14, 15], that secondary intervention is best pursued after about a week. The advantages are that this period of time allows for natural hemostasis, improvement in any corneal edema, occurrence or at least more inducible posterior vitreous separation, liquefaction of hemorrhage, and optimal resources for surgery, while still preempting the proliferative process demonstrated by the experimental models cited above.

3.5 Choroidal Hemorrhage

This is usually incidental to other ocular traumas. While principles relevant to spontaneous choroidal hemorrhage are applicable, the setting of the hemorrhage usually makes this more of an incidental problem. The scope of the surgery to drain the hemorrhage is commonly determined by other features of the injury; more often than not, the choroidal hemorrhage is drained in conjunction with other features of repair. However, as for spontaneous choroidal hemorrhages, those that do not approach the position of apposition are usually self-limited and require no treatment. If there is apposition that does not show signs of spontaneous abatement within a week, drainage should be strongly considered [16].

As a general rule, the hemorrhage clots within minutes, as evidenced by the difficulty of trying to drain acute choroidal hemorrhages occurring during surgery, but after 7–10 days, the clot retracts, allowing liquefaction of most of the mass of the hemorrhage; at that time drainage is almost trivial. This circumstance can be managed with a sclerotomy in the meridian of the hemorrhage. The ideal location is to place this anterior to the ora serrata, but it must be within the extent of the hemorrhage.

3.6 Traumatic Macular Holes

Macular holes (MH) do occur in association with blunt trauma, probably from a forceful coup–contrecoup force via the vitreous insertion at the fovea, although some make note of traumatic MHs may occur from breakthrough subretinal hemorrhage into VH at the fovea. As with the epidemiology of ocular trauma in general, these are more common in a younger age group (young adults, but also children – eyes with firm vitreous attachment at the posterior pole) and with a male predominance. The size of the MH can be larger than their idiopathic counterpart. The treatment and management are not distinguished from idiopathic cases, but the success rate is generally poorer and may bespeak a slightly altered pathogenic mechanism. The same surgical techniques as for idiopathic macular holes have been reported to yield similar results [17–20], although it is this author's experience that the macular holes are usually larger and perhaps, this combined with more photoreceptor disintegration from the commotio retinae injury, the prognosis is poorer.

3.7 Traumatic Optic Neuropathy

This is a common consequence of blunt trauma, occurring in about 5% of head trauma [21]. Severe blunt force may rarely lead to optic nerve avulsion [22]. Direct trauma as from a penetrating object is a common cause, but many indirect causes of optic neuropathy may also follow from a traumatic injury such as bony fractures where the optic nerve exits the cranium or due to compartment syndrome secondary to retrobulbar bleeding [23]. There is no specific treatment for traumatic optic neuropathy except to recognize possible secondary compression causes, but it is commonly not recognized until irreversible damage has occurred. The value of pulsed systemic corticosteroids has not been shown to be transferrable from its idiopathic, inflammatory counterpart [24, 25].

3.8 Categories of Injury: Open Versus Closed Globe Injury

The extreme heterogeneity of trauma effects can most meaningfully be categorized as eyes suffering blunt trauma versus eyes sustaining penetrating trauma. There is much overlap with a categorization as open globe (more commonly sharp induced) versus closed globe (more commonly blunt) injuries.

While clearly the target component most affected is what determines prognosis, and even treatment strategy, generally penetrating trauma causes more of its effects local to the injury with fewer distant effects. Generally, the force of injury is less with penetrating injuries, and the sharp incisional injury lends itself to a better prognosis of treatment. On the other hand, blunt injury more commonly induces primary injury to distant targets such as the ON, macula, and vitreous base.

As mentioned above, the nature and size of the injury are one of the most important prognostic factors [8].

3.9 Secondary Management of Trauma Including Retinal Detachment

As alluded to above, a violation of the vitreous base (or structures behind the ora serrata) regardless of the extent of the injury calls for at least a prompt intervention, with the idea of minimizing the spread or even precluding the occurrence of cicatricial retinal detachment. Post-traumatic proliferative vitreoretinopathy (PVR) is the demon that prevents success in many cases of ocular trauma, especially with open globe injuries and those with secondary retinal detachment [26].

The techniques for treating cases with PVR and retinal detachment are essentially the same as for treatment of complex retinal detachment.

While techniques for managing complex retinal detachments are changing, with fewer proponents of scleral buckling, this author favors using a scleral buckle whenever the vitreous base has been violated. The scleral buckle offers neutralization of cicatricial traction, whether already present or if soon to be present. Retinal incarceration is a common circumstance after primary closure and represents an ominous prerequisite for further traction. Membranes are usually not manifest until a few weeks post injury and are usually commensurate with retinal detachment formation. Maximal removal of media opacities, maximal vitreous removal, and neutralization of traction with the scleral buckling are the earliest steps. If there are epiretinal membranes that are mature enough to peel, these should also be removed. Broad application of laser is important whether or not there is already a rhegmatogenous situation; however, judicious use of laser is urged or else there might be an exacerbation of the inflammation that drives the PVR process.

If there is a rhegmatogenous component to the retinal detachment, intraocular tamponade is necessary. The same considerations governing the choice of tamponading agents apply to the trauma eye with retinal detachment. Relatively localized pathology might be considered for intraocular gas only, the duration of which is further selected contingent upon the assessed severity. Silicone oil is a valuable tool that is generally reserved for more severe cases due to its potential complications and the need to consider a future operation for removal.

Ancillary considerations pertain to management of anterior segment injuries concurrent with repair of secondary retinal detachment. The threshold to remove a crystalline lens should be low, as the advantages of improved visibility and the simplification of reducing the eye to a unicameral eye are great; optical rehabilitation can be performed at a later time if the repair has been otherwise favorable. Similarly, repair of iridodialysis or pupillary damage can be effected when more severe complications are in hand. The disadvantage of possible silicone oil prolapse is small compared to these advantages, as generally this is manageable either in the clinic or with a return to the operating room.

Later complications such as corneal decompensation or glaucoma may require partnering with those respective specialists, again once those objectives are rendered relevant by virtue of stabilizing the posterior segment.

Illustrative Cases

1. Choroidal hemorrhage (Fig. 3.1)

   A 75-year-old male fell causing blunt trauma to his right eye. He was seen 1 week later for consultation with vision of hand motions. There was a right afferent pupillary defect. Examination disclosed an anterior chamber intraocular lens, minimal vitreous hemorrhage, and a high, nearly appositional choroidal hemorrhage that was higher temporally. There was no scleral rupture. There was questionable retinal detachment, but this was thought to be secondary to the choroidal hemorrhage since it occurred in a limited fashion at the posterior base of the choroid (Fig. 3.1). The ultrasound test demonstrated liquefied choroidal hemorrhage.

   He underwent surgery to drain the hemorrhage. The conjunctiva was opened temporally, and a circumferential sclerotomy was performed just anterior to the muscle insertions. Copious dark red blood egressed. The sclerotomy was not sutured. A scleral buckle was not placed and a vitrectomy was not performed.

   Postoperatively, the retina remained reattached and the vitreous hemorrhage cleared completely. The residual choroidal gradually resolved as did the subretinal fluid. Cystoid macular edema occurred within the first month but responded, ultimately, to intravitreal triamcinolone. There was increasing corneal edema that required a DSEK. The visual acuity was 20/80 18 months after the initial injury.

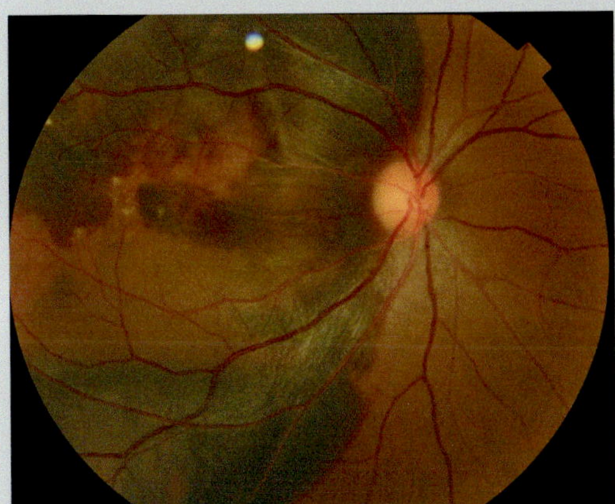

Fig. 3.1 Photograph showing diffuse subretinal hemorrhage one weeks following vitrectomy and drainage of choroidal hemorrhage induced by blunt trauma. There is a low, residual choroidal hemorrhage in the far temporal periphery (not illustrated), but this is markedly diminished

One might have considered a more conservative approach with continued observation, but due to the height of the choroidal hemorrhage, the profound visual loss, and the patient's strong motivation to intercede at that point in time, the drainage was performed as described. Another consideration for the approach would have considered a primary vitrectomy in conjunction with the drainage. In retrospect, the vitreous hemorrhage and subretinal fluid (which seemed to have been secondary to the choroidal hemorrhage) resolved without consequence. The corneal decompensation likely was attributable in part to the trauma but probably was largely due to preexisting compromise from what was, evidently, a complicated previous cataract extraction.

2. Timing of vitrectomy after primary repair
A 29-year-old male was involved in an altercation and sustained an injury to his left eye from some broken glass. The visual acuity was hand motions, and there was not an afferent pupillary defect. There was a laceration evident that extended from about 3 mm posterior to the temporal limbus posteriorly. The cornea was fairly clear and there did not appear to be any lens rupture, but there was blood lining the posterior lens surface. There was moderate vitreous hemorrhage which blocked the view posteriorly. An X-ray did not depict any intraocular foreign body. A primary closure with silk sutures was affected the next morning. The posterior extent of the laceration was about 3 mm behind the line of the muscle insertions.

One week later, the visual acuity was 1/200 with still moderate vitreous hemorrhage. The ultrasound test did not show retinal detachment. A vitrectomy was performed in conjunction with an encircling scleral buckling procedure with a 240 band and a lensectomy (preserving the peripheral anterior capsule). The visual acuity had improved to 20/40 by 2 months postoperatively (with aphakic correction). A secondary PC IOL was planned.

In this case there are several points of controversy. Whenever the vitreous base has been affected by a rupture or laceration (Fig. 3.2a), the risk of subsequent retinal detachment is high (as the experimental and clinical studies cited above have demonstrated). While it would have been very reasonable to perform the vitrectomy commensurate with the laceration repair, this surgeon prefers a staged approach about 10 days later so that the posterior vitreous detachment could either occur or more easily be induced. Such trauma more commonly involves a younger population without preexisting vitreous separation. Removal of the posterior hyaloid is important to minimize postoperative cellular proliferation that could lead to retinal detachment. Placement of an encircling scleral buckle neutralizes some of the cicatricial vitreous changes consequent to such an injury (Fig. 3.2b). The lens was removed in this case to facilitate maximal vitreous base removal and to maximize visualization. The peripheral anterior capsule was preserved to allow future placement of a posterior chamber IOL into the sulcus.

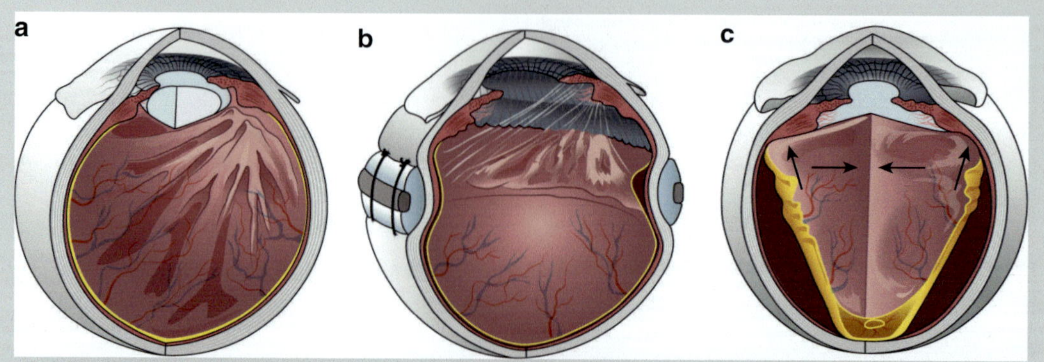

Fig. 3.2 Schematic depicting vitreous traction towards anterior laceration site (**a**). Vitrectomy and scleral buckling procedure were performed (**b**). If vitreous traction is not addressed early, secondary "anterior loop" traction may ensue causing severe cicatricial changes (**c**) (Permission from Michels RG, et al. Retinal Detachment. CV Mosby 1990)

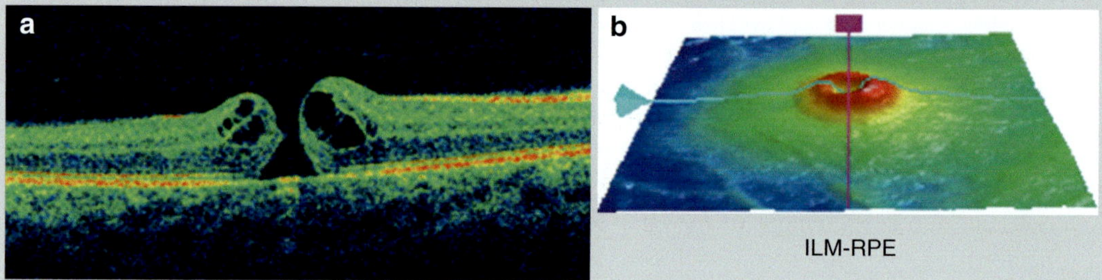

Fig. 3.3 Optical coherence tomograph of a traumatically induced full-thickness macular hole (**a**) with the map showing elevation and thickening of adjacent foveal tissue (**b**)

While there might be debate about whether the vitrectomy should be done concurrent with the primary closure or up to 10 days later, there is uniform agreement that waiting in the hopes that the vitreous hemorrhage would clear, or only if it did not clear after several weeks, is contraindicated due to the expectation that contraction of the vitreous base during that time would lead to a complex retinal detachment (Fig. 3.2c).

3. Traumatic macular hole (Fig. 3.3)

   A 32-year-old male was struck by a random rock on the right side of his head and brow. One week later, he realized loss of central vision. He was seen 2 weeks later with 20/80 due to a small macular hole (Fig. 3.3). The lens was clear and stable. The only other definite sign of trauma was a self-healed retinal dialysis inferotemporally, but there might have been mild RPE disturbance in the 1-disk-diameter radius around the fovea suggesting previous commotio retinae. There was a posterior vitreous detachment.

   A vitrectomy with ILM peel and fluid–gas exchange was performed. No chromodyes or triamcinolone was used. Medium-acting gas was used since the patient had to fly home as soon as possible.

   A concern in traumatic macular holes is the possibility of permanent visual loss due to collateral injury, such as cataract, commotio retinae, or optic neuropathy. Treatment of traumatic macular holes is identical in approach as for idiopathic macular holes.

4. Blunt trauma (Fig. 3.4)

   A 16-year-old was struck by a paintball after removing his protective eyewear after completing a "war games" contest. He had sudden and severe loss of vision. He was seen the next day with recorded light perception vision and intraocular pressure of 26 mmHg. There was a moderately hazy view to the posterior pole due to some vitreous hemorrhage. The media had improved sufficiently by weeks later to allow view of a submacular hemorrhage (Fig. 3.4). This cleared spontaneously over the next 3 months yielding 20/15 visual acuity. There were no other collateral injuries, for example, to the vitreous base or lens.

Subretinal hemorrhage itself is not generally an indication for surgical intervention since, especially in young patients, there is a good capacity for spontaneous resolution, as occurred in this patient [27]. This case does demonstrate the importance of compulsive use of protective eyewear in this growing recreational pastime of paintball contests [28].

5. Secondary RD after trauma (SB, SO, options for management – like PVR: retinotomy, lens, etc.) (Fig. 3.5)
A 49-year-old man suffered an injury to his left eye when a tennis ball hit his eye directly. He had a su dden and severe loss of vision. He was seen the next day with vision of 3/200 and a moderate circulating hyphema; there did not appear to be any retinal detachment by ophthalmoscopy (limited by media opacities) or

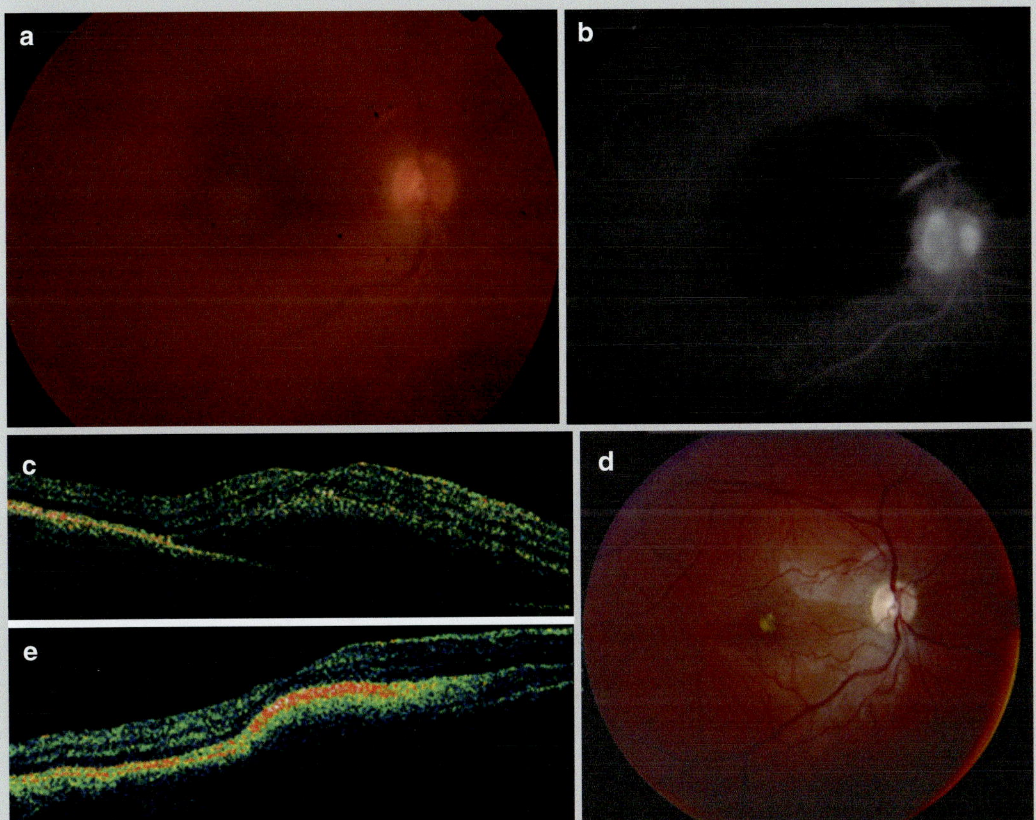

Fig. 3.4 Fundus photograph of submacular hemorrhage (**a**), better appreciated for its extent on the red free photography (**b**). The OCT shows the subretinal hemorrhage (**c**). Three weeks later the fundus (**d**) and OCT (**e**) have improved

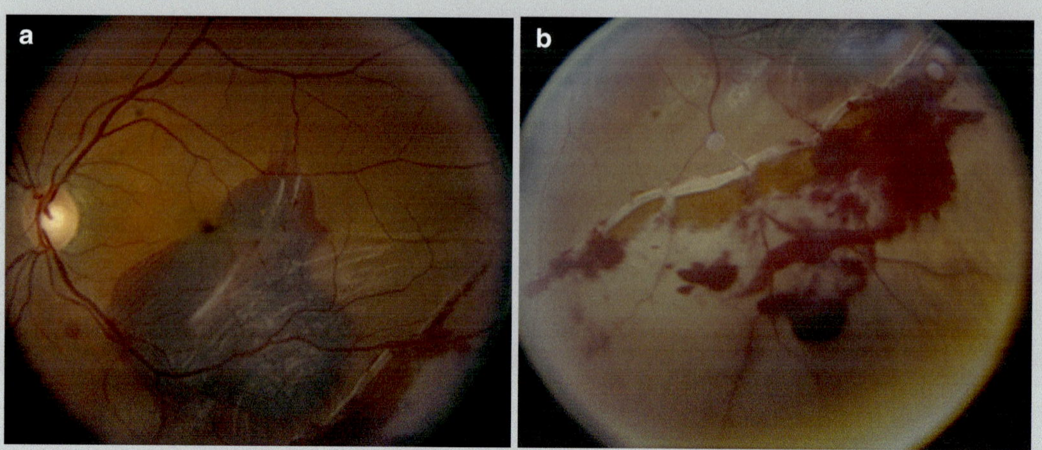

Fig. 3.5 Fundus photograph shows subretinal hemorrhage with shallow subretinal fluid (**a**). Views further inferotemporally show the large break with adjacent preretinal hemorrhage and bridging retinal vessels (**b**)

ultrasound examination. One week later, the hyphema had cleared sufficiently to allow detection of a subretinal hemorrhage underlying the fovea and extending inferiorly (Fig. 3.5). There was a 3-clock-hour tear with bridging vessels in the mid-periphery associated with hemorrhage and subretinal fluid extending around the tear and inferiorly.

A vitrectomy was performed with the use of endolaser and silicone oil due to the extent of the retinal tear. A scleral buckle was not used in this case due to the exclusively posterior nature of the retinal pathology. The vitreous was avulsed temporally but still attached at the optic nerve head, so the posterior hyaloid was induced to be completely detached. The subretinal hemorrhage was partially removed during surgery; the remainder resolved spontaneously during the next several weeks. It became apparent that the hemorrhage was from a limited, subjacent choroidal rupture. The silicone oil was removed 6 months later. The final vision was 20/50.

In this case silicone oil might not have been necessary, but due to the concern for later epiretinal membrane proliferation, it was chosen over the use of a gas tamponade. It is also questionable as to whether the subretinal hemorrhage should have been evacuated, but since it was not simply a thin layer and since it was so readily available through the nearby tear, it was aspirated with a satisfying result. In contrast to subretinal hemorrhages in association with choroidal neovascular membranes which commonly involve the sub-RPE space and RPE denudation when evacuated, subretinal membranes due to blunt trauma more commonly are confined to the subretinal space. However, as in these cases, a choroidal rupture is a common source and may itself be the limiting factor in the visual acuity.

Clinical Pearls

1. Vitreous hemorrhage after trauma, unless trivial, should not be managed conservatively by extended observation, as its very presence (especially after penetrating trauma) augurs a poor prognosis.
2. Globe ruptures or lacerations involving the vitreous base usually provoke substantial cellular proliferation into the vitreous base with subsequent contraction. A timely scleral buckle combined with maximal vitrectomy can avert retinal consequences of this.
3. Traumatic macular holes are generally treated in the same manner as idiopathic macular holes but, due to their typically larger size and collateral injuries, usually have a poorer anatomic and visual result.
4. Preservation of peripheral anterior lens capsule is an effective means of gaining access to peripheral retina and vitreous while preserving opportunity for visual rehabilitation with PC IOL placement into the ciliary sulcus (with proper adjustment for the IOL power calculation).
5. Sequential examinations are recommended in cases of apparently closed globe injury, as subsequent vitreoretinal changes may occur which, if undetected early, may lead to severe late visual complications.

References

1. de Juan E, Hickingbotham Jr D. Refinements in microinstrumentation for vitreous surgery. Am J Ophthalmol. 1990;109:218–20.
2. Topping TM, Abrams GW, Machemer R. Experimental double-perforating injury of the posterior segment in rabbit eyes: the natural history of intraocular proliferation. Arch Ophthalmol. 1979;97:735–42.
3. Abrams GW, Topping TM, Machemer R. Vitrectomy for injury: the effect on intraocular proliferation following perforation of the posterior segment of the rabbit eye. Arch Ophthalmol. 1979;97:743–8.
4. Cleary PE, Ryan SJ. Vitrectomy in penetrating eye injury: results of a controlled trial of vitrectomy in an experimental posterior penetrating eye injury in the rhesus monkey. Arch Ophthalmol. 1981;99:287–92.
5. Gregor Z, Ryan SJ. Complete and core vitrectomies in the treatment of experimental posterior penetrating eye injury in the rhesus monkey. I. Clinical features. Arch Ophthalmol. 1983;101:441–5.
6. Gregor Z, Ryan SJ. Complete and core vitrectomies in the treatment of experimental posterior penetrating eye injury in the rhesus monkey. II. Histologic features. Arch Ophthalmol. 1983;101:446–50.
7. De Juan Jr E, Sternberg Jr P, Michels RG, Auer C. Evaluation of vitrectomy in penetrating ocular trauma: a case control study. Arch Ophthalmol. 1984;102:1160–3.
8. Sternberg Jr P, de Juan E, Michaels RG. Multivariate analysis of prognostic factors in penetrating ocular injuries. Am J Ophchalmol. 1984;98:467–72.
9. Hutton WL, Fuller DG. Factors influencing final visual results in severely injured eyes. Am J Ophrhalmol. 1984;97:715–22.
10. Gilbert CM, Soong HK, Hirst LW. A two year prospective study of penetrating ocular trauma at the Wilmer Ophthalmological Institute. Ann Ophthalmol. 1987;19:104–6.
11. Coleman DJ. Early vitrectomy in the management of the severely traumatized eye. Am J Ophthalmol. 1982;93:543–51.
12. Green WR. The uveal tract. In: Spencer WI-I, editor. Ophthalmic pathology. Philadelphia: WB Saunders; 1986.
13. Lubin JR, Albert DM, Weinstein M. Sixty five years of sympathetic ophthalmia. A clinicopathologic review of 105 cases (1913–1978). Ophthalmology. 1980;87:109–21.
14. Conway BP, Michels RG. Vitrectomy techniques in the management of selected penetrating ocular injuries. Ophthalmology. 1978;85:560.
15. Michels RG. Vitrectomy methods in penetrating ocular trauma. Ophthalmology. 1980;87:629.
16. Pakravan M, Yazdani S, Afroozifar M, Kouhestani N, Ghassami M, Shahshahan M. An alternative approach for management of delayed suprachoroidal hemorrhage after glaucoma procedures. J Glaucoma. 2014;23:37–40.
17. Garcia-Arumi J, Corcostegui B, Cavero L, Sararols L. The role of vitreoretinal surgery in the treatment of posttraumatic macular hole. Retina. 1997;17:372–7.
18. Barreau E, Massin P, Paques M, Santiago PY, Gaudric A. Surgical treatment of posttraumatic macular holes. J Fran d Ophtalmol. 1997;20(6):423–9.
19. Madreperla SA, Benetz BA. Formation and treatment of a traumatic macular hole. Arch Ophthalmol. 1997;115(9):1210–1.
20. de Bustros S. Vitreous surgery for traumatic macular hole. Retina. 1996;16(5):451–2.

21. Gjerris F. Traumatic lesions of the visual pathways. In: Vinken PJ, Bruyn GW, editors. Handbook of critical neurology, vol. 24. Amsterdam: North-Holland Pub Co; 1976. p. 27–57.
22. Williams DF, Williams GA, Abrams GW, et al. Evulsion of the retina associated with optic nerve evulsion. Am J Ophthalmol. 1987;104:5–9.
23. Steinsapir KD, Goldberg RA. Traumatic optic neuropathy. Surv Ophthalmol. 1994;38:487–518.
24. Spoor TC, Hartel WC, Lensink DB, Wilkinson MJ. Treatment of traumatic optic neuropathy with corticosteroids. AM J Opthalmol. 1990;110:665–9.
25. Mauriello JA, Deluca J, Kreiger A, et al. Management of traumatic optic neuropathy: a study of 23 patients. Br J Ophthalmol. 1992;76:349–52.
26. Cardillo JA, Stout JT, LaBree L, et al. Post-traumatic proliferative vitreoretinopathy. Epidemiol. 1997;104(7):1166–73.
27. Berrocal MH, Lewis ML, Flynn Jr HW. Variations in the clinical course of submacular hemorrhage. Am J Ophthalmol. 1996;122(4):486–93.
28. Alliman KJ, Smiddy WE, Banta J, Quershi Y, Miller DM, Schiffman JC. Ocular trauma and visual outcome secondary to paintball projectiles. Am J Ophthalmol. 2009;147(2):239–42.

4 Intraocular Foreign Bodies

Hua Yan, Jiaxing Wang, Caiyun You, and Xiangda Meng

4.1 Introduction

Intraocular foreign body (IOFB), a kind of ophthalmic emergency, accounts for about 6 % of the ocular trauma and is commonly seen in young male [1]. The foreign bodies not only cause mechanical damage but also bring pathogenic microorganisms into the eyes, leading to endophthalmitis, which seriously affects the prognosis of visual acuity. These make IOFBs to be one of the leading causes of monocular blindness. The longer foreign bodies stay in the eyes, the greater damage they make. For those reasons, early diagnosis and treatment of IOFBs is important.

In this chapter, we described the clinical characteristics and treatment of IOFBs. A variety of IOFB cases such as anterior chamber foreign body, retinal foreign body, and giant IOFB were presented. Hot topics in the current understanding of IOFB and consensuses and controversies were thoroughly discussed.

H. Yan, MD, PhD (✉) • J. Wang, MD
C. You, MD, PhD • X. Meng, MD, PhD
Department of Ophthalmology, Tianjin Medical University General Hospital, Tianjin, China
e-mail: phuayan2000@163.com

4.2 Management Differences Between Types of IOFBs

Intraocular foreign body, a kind of ophthalmic emergency, accounts for about 6 % of the ocular trauma and is commonly seen in young male [1]. The foreign bodies not only cause mechanical damage but also bring pathogenic microorganisms into the eyes, leading to endophthalmitis, which seriously affects the prognosis of visual acuity. These make IOFBs to be one of the leading causes of monocular blindness. The longer foreign bodies stay in the eyes, the greater damage they make. For those reasons, early diagnosis and treatment of IOFBs is important.

4.2.1 Classification

According to their properties, IOFBs can be classified into metallic foreign bodies (active metals like iron, copper, etc. and inert metals) and nonmetallic foreign bodies (stable foreign bodies like glasses and unstable foreign bodies like wood). Different types of foreign bodies lead to different pathophysiological process. Metallic foreign bodies, especially active metals, may make severe damage to the eyes within a short time due to its toxicity. Long time retain of active metals in the eye can cause siderosis or chalcosis, with poor prognosis. Wooden foreign bodies have a great chance of causing endophthalmitis.

H. Yan (ed.), *Mechanical Ocular Trauma*, DOI 10.1007/978-981-10-2150-3_4

Distinction between magnetic and nonmagnetic IOFBs is important for surgical options. Vitrectomy is the only way to remove nonmagnetic IOFBs. However, magnetic IOFBs can be removed by a magnet or vitrectomy.

4.2.2 Clinical Manifestation

Clinical manifestation can be extremely complicated. It varies depending on the location of the wound track and retaining time of the foreign bodies in the eyes. Anterior segment foreign bodies may just lead to the changes of anterior chamber, iris, ciliary body, and lens. However, foreign bodies in vitreous cavity or posterior ocular wall may cause severe damage to the whole eye. Long term of IOFBs may increase the risk of sight-threatening endophthalmitis.

Common symptoms and signs are listed below:

- Symptoms: pain, decreased vision
- Signs:
  - Wound track: conjunctiva, cornea, and sclera
  - Changes of anterior chamber: shallow anterior chamber, the absence of anterior chamber, deep anterior chamber, hyphema, hypopyon, and aqueous flare
  - Pupil distortion: pupil turn toward the penetration site
  - Changes of lens: lens opacity, rupture of lens capsule, and lens subluxation and dislocation
  - Traumatic cyclodialysis
  - Vitreous opacity
  - Changes of ocular fundus: retinal/choroidal tear or detachment, fundus hemorrhage, and intraocular foreign body
  - Prolapse of eye contents
  - Decreased intraocular pressure

4.2.3 Diagnosis and Localization

Direct or indirect fundus ophthalmoscope and fundus preset lens can help locate the IOFBs in patients with clear refractive media most intuitively. However, more often, the refractive media of the injured eye is muddy. In this case, imageological examination will be requested.

X-ray X-ray examination is a traditional diagnostic method of IOFBs and is easy to operate. Patients should receive X-ray examination in two directions (an AP view and a lateral view). Foreign bodies with high density, such as metals, stones, and glasses, can be clearly depicted by X-ray. However, the eyeball cannot be shown on plain film. Therefore, the localization of IOFBs should be dependent on the locator, quite restrict. Image of an IOFB on X-ray is shown in Fig. 4.1

CT Computed tomography (CT), with its high resolution and positive rate comparing to X-ray, is considered to be the gold standard for the diagnosis of IOFBs [2], especially for diagnosing small metallic foreign bodies and nonmetallic foreign bodies. CT helps display the structure of

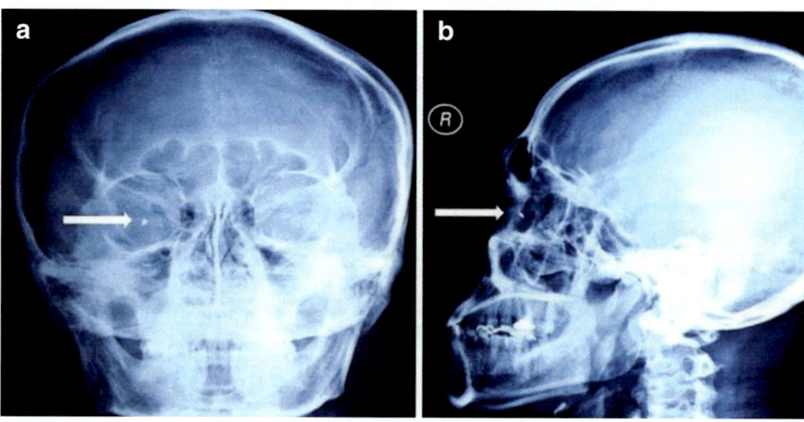

Fig. 4.1 An intraocular foreign body on X-ray. (**a**) Coronal scan; (**b**) lateral scan. *White arrow* shows the IOFB

the eyeball and can clearly localize the anatomical position of the foreign body. Furthermore, ophthalmologists can estimate the nature of the foreign bodies according to their CT values and artifacts. Both the plain scan and coronal scan should be taken for accurately locating the IOFBs. Characteristics and images of different IOFBs on CT are shown in Table 4.1 and Figs. 4.2, 4.3, and 4.4. The normal CT values of intraocular structures are shown in Table 4.2.

MRI Magnetic foreign body is the contraindication of magnetic resonance imaging (MRI) examination because its translocation under MRI may cause second damage to the eye. An MRI examination is of value when there is a high suspicion of nonmetallic IOFBs, especially wooden foreign body with a negative CT image (Fig. 4.5) [3]. Nonmetallic IOFBs show low signal on both T1W1 and T2W1 sequences. Vitreous and aqueous humor shows low signal on T1W1 sequence and high signal on T2W1 sequence. Nonmetallic IOFBs are easily recognized on T2W1 sequence.

A/B-Scan Ultrasound Under B-scan examination, the appearance of IOFBs could be intraocular strong echoes with posterior acoustic shadow (Fig. 4.6). Combined with single high waves in A-scan, IOFBs can be accurately diagnosed.

Table 4.1 Characteristics of different IOFBs on CT

Nature of IOFBs	Characteristics
Metallic IOFBs	High-density images (CT values, 1000–2000 HU) Artifacts
Stone, glass, bone, silicon oil, etc.	High-density images (CT values, >300 HU) No artifacts
Plants	Slightly hyperdensity, mixed density, or low-density images No artifacts

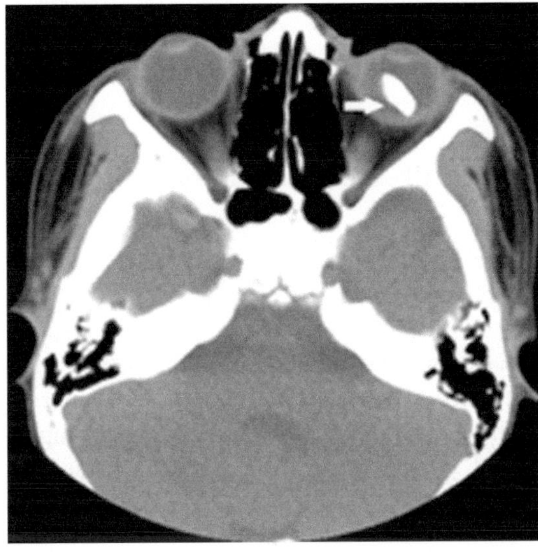

Fig. 4.3 A glass foreign body on CT imaging (*white arrow*)

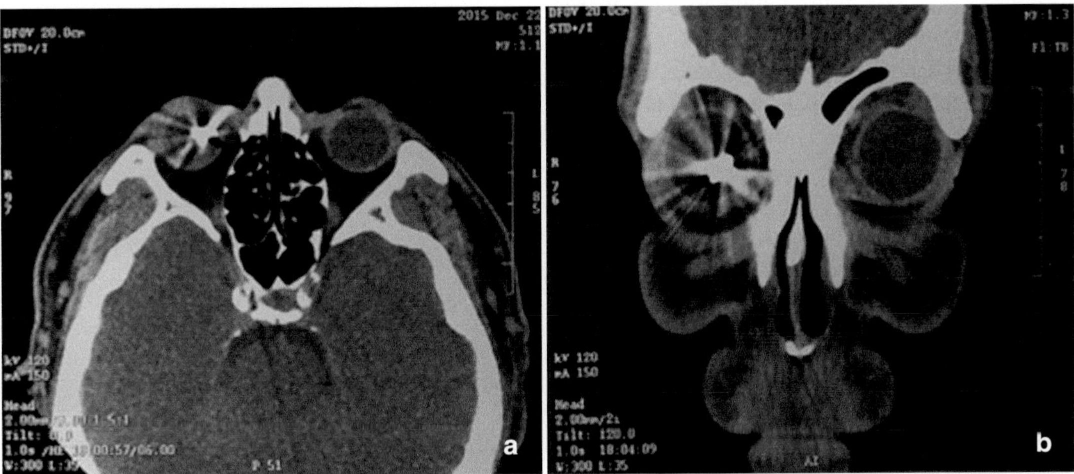

Fig. 4.2 An iron foreign body on CT. *Left*: plain scan; *right*: coronal scan

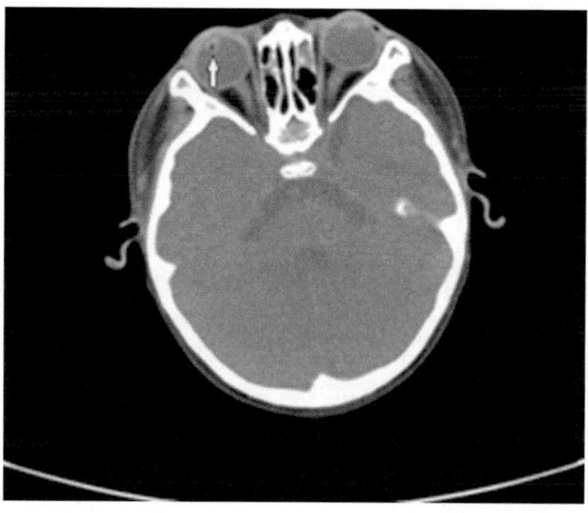

Fig. 4.4 A plant foreign body on CT imaging (*white arrow*)

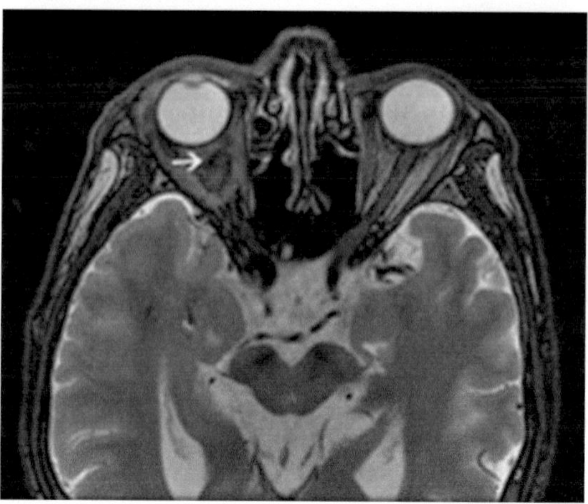

Fig. 4.5 An orbital wooden foreign body on MRI (*white arrow*)

Table 4.2 CT values of intraocular structures

Lens	70–80 HU
Vitreous	0–10 HU
Bone	>400 HU

What should be pointed out is that A/B-scan is not suitable for patients suffering severe traumatic eyeball rupture or combined with complex eyelid laceration before the eye is closed by surgery.

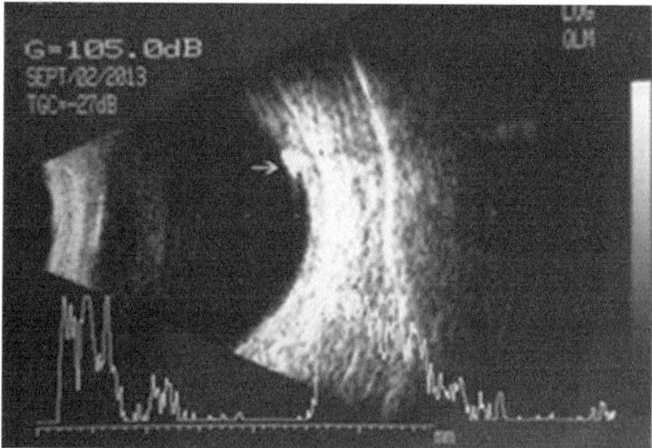

Fig. 4.6 An intraocular foreign body on A/B ultrasound (*white arrow*)

UBM Ultrasound biomicroscopy (UBM) examination plays an important role in showing anterior segment IOFBs (Fig. 4.7), especially for tiny foreign bodies (<1 mm) which located in the anterior chamber, equator lentis, or near the ciliary body. These kinds of foreign bodies have little influence on visual acuity in the early days after injury and can be hardly found by routine ocular exams. All kinds of foreign bodies could appear strong echoes without posterior acoustic shadow in UBM, no matter it is metallic or nonmetallic foreign bodies.

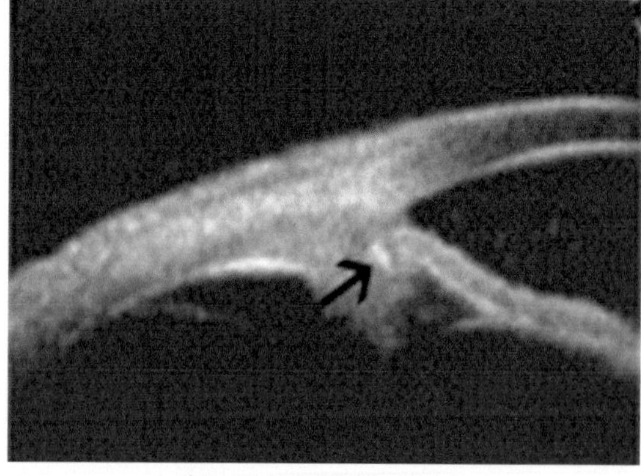

Fig. 4.7 An intraocular foreign body on UBM (*black arrow*)

Treatment When an IOFB is suspected, the injured eye should be bandaged sterilely and immediately. Anti-infection and anti-tetanus therapies should be performed before the emergency surgery.

The purpose of emergency surgery is to close the wound of the eye, reconstruct the anterior chamber, recover, and maintain the intraocular pressure immediately. For IOFBs, they should be removed as early as possible because of the potential risk of endophthalmitis and its toxicity [4–6]. However, timing of IOFB removal is controversial presently [7, 8]. Magnetic foreign bodies located in the clear anterior vitreous cavity can be attracted out by using a magnet at pars plana sclerotomy site. Foreign bodies in the anterior chamber can be precisely extracted by using different intraocular forceps according to the size of the IOFBs. All kinds of IOFBs can be removed precisely using vitrectomy no matter what characters of foreign body and where the foreign body located in the posterior segment. Meanwhile, the vitreous inflammatory factors, vitreous hemorrhage, IOFB-induced proliferative vitreoretinopathy (PVR), and other disorders in the posterior segment can be completely treated during vitrectomy.

Some complicated cases need secondary surgery to help with the reconstruction of the intraocular structure.

4.3 Illustrative Case(s) of Intraocular Foreign Bodies

Location and size of the IOFBs may result in vision loss independently, regardless of the type of injury and characteristic of the foreign body. The following cases illustrate the IOFBs involved in various parts of the injured eyes and some specific cases. According to recent studies, 58 % IOFB locates in posterior segment, 13–24 % in anterior segment, 7–10 % in lens, 25–48 % in vitreous, 16–44 % in retina, 52 % in both retina and choroid, and 0–15 % subretinally [9] (Figs. 4.8, 4.9, 4.10, and 4.11).

4.3.1 Giant IOFB

A 45-year-old man presented with a 12-h history of a transverse irregular corneal laceration from 3 o'clock to 9 o'clock position with iris and vitreous prolapse after being hit by a piece of iron in the left eye. The wound was closed by primary repair of corneoscleral laceration on the first presentation day. His left eye had best corrected visual acuity (BCVA) of no light perception. Slit-lamp examination presented chemosis, corneal edema, disappearance of anterior chamber, intraocular hemorrhage, and traumatic cataract. Fundus details were not clear due to severe vitreous hemorrhage. B-scan ultrasonography identified a hyperechogenic shadowing that was concerning for an IOFB (Fig. 4.11a). Computed tomography showed a metallic IOFB in the vitreous (Fig. 4.11b). Examination of the right eye was unremarkable.

Eight days after primary repair, we removed the IOFB through an open-sky corneal incision followed by a 23-gauge pars plana vitrectomy (PPV) using a TPK. Firstly, the irrigation-aspiration was performed for removing the exudates and hemorrhage in the anterior chamber (Fig. 4.11c). Then injured cornea was excised using a 7.25-mm trephine (Fig. 4.11d), and the corneal graft was protected by a viscoelastic material and kept in a humid container. After the inflammation tissue of the anterior segment was removed, the IOFB appeared and was separated completely from all surrounding tissues. Then it was grasped with forceps and extracted through the open-sky corneal incision (Fig. 4.11e, f). PPV was performed by using a TPK which

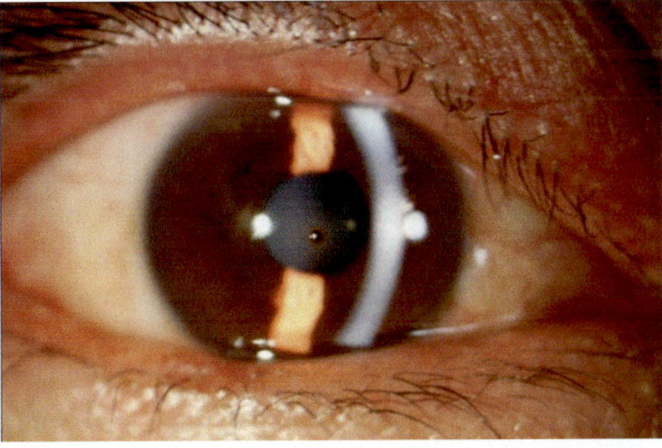

Fig. 4.8 An iron foreign body imbedded in the superficial corneal stroma, with rust ring and corneal edema surrounded. The slit illumination is used in the appreciation of the exact depth of the foreign body

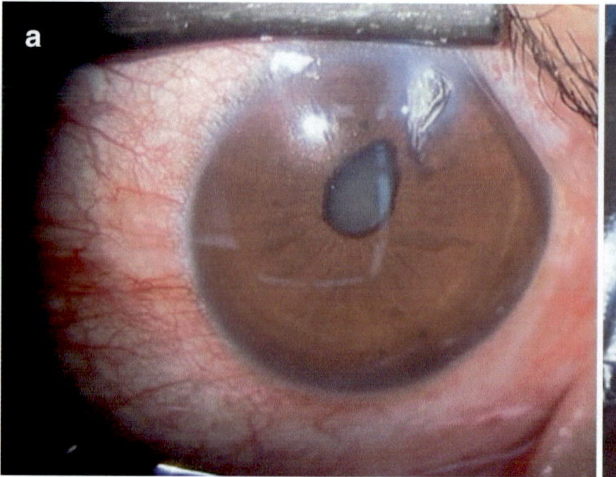

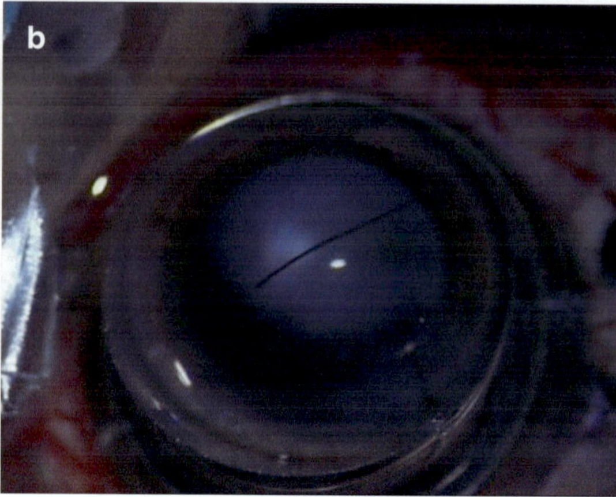

Fig. 4.9 (**a**) An eye suffered from a penetrating injury including cornea, iris, and lens. An irregular metal IOFB was embedded in the cornea, iris, and lens at 1 o'clock position (*black arrow*). It has caused the pupil deformation, iris laceration, and focal opacity of the lens. Vision was seriously impaired. (**b**) An eye suffered from a penetrating injury. An eyelash was located in the anterior chamber and was removed from the anterior chamber during vitrectomy. The removed eyelash is shown on the contact lens (*white arrow*). The eyelash might bring microorganisms to the eye and cause severe endophthalmitis

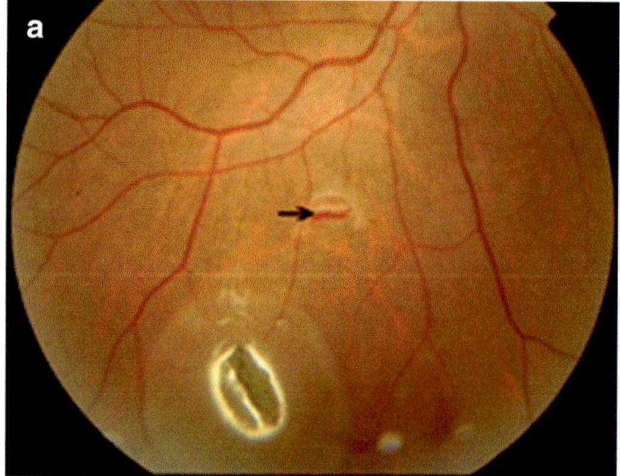

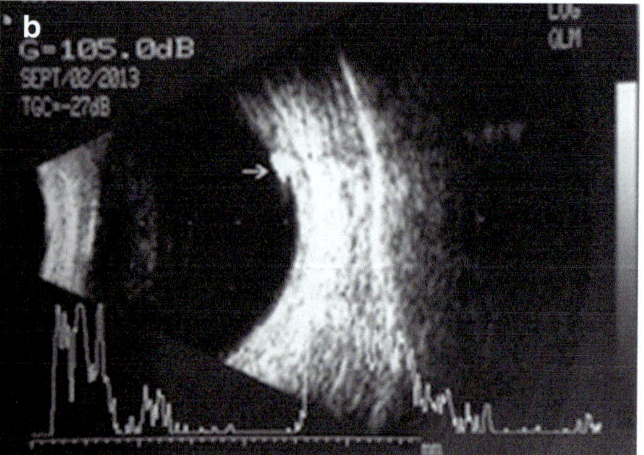

Fig. 4.10 (**a**) An iron IOFB was embedded in the inferior-temporal retina. The obvious retina edema was seen just surrounding the IOFB, which might eventually develop to retinal detachment. A crescented retinal hole was located above the IOFB with tiny retinal hemorrhage (*black arrow*). It is suspected that the IOFB dropped on the retina resulting in the crescented retinal hole and then bumped to the fixed position of the retina. The best corrected visual acuity (BCVA) was 20/50. (**b**) B-scan ultrasonography demonstrated the IOFB located in the retina (*white arrow*)

included membrane peeling, use of perfluorocarbon liquids, photocoagulation, and silicone oil filling. At the end, the patient's injured corneal graft was sutured back with 10-0 Vicryl suture.

Removal of a giant IOFB by the traditional technique usually requires a relatively large sclerotomy which can damage the ciliary body and peripheral retina because it is difficult to precisely locate the position of the IOFB and fully expose the posterior globe wall [10]. Similarly, removal of a giant IOFB through the corneal limbus incision combined with PPV also has their limitations. Kunikata et al. [11] showed two cases of 25-gauge microincision vitrectomy surgery for removal of large IOFB through the 2.4- or 3.0-mm corneal incision. However, this technique is best suited to long slender smooth foreign body and cannot be used for giant and irregular-shaped foreign body.

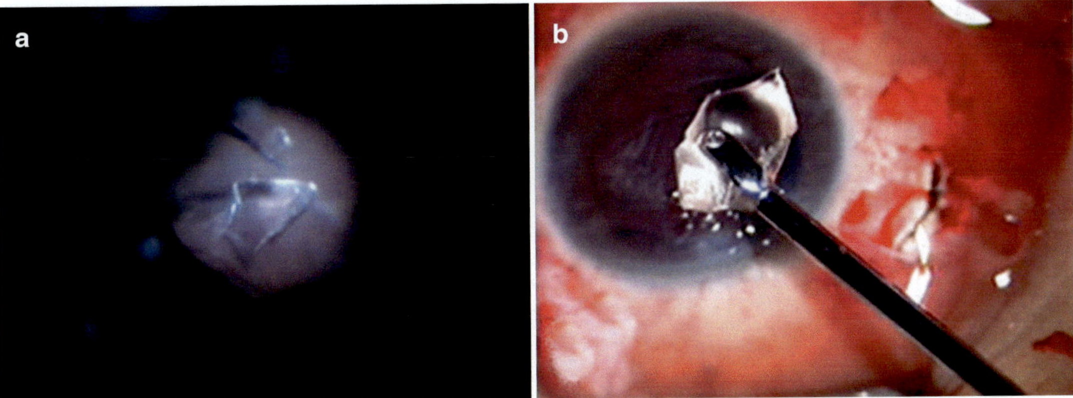

Fig. 4.11 (a) An irregular glass IOFB was lying on the retinal surface. It has induced a fibrinous reaction around the IOFB. (b) The IOFB was successfully removed by enlarging the sclerotomy

In this case, open-sky approach presents the following advantages. Firstly, it allows easy and direct access to the giant IOFB, so that the surgical damage to retina, ciliary body, or other ocular structures can be avoided. Secondly, the surgeon can grasp the giant IOFB easily and steadily with forceps, which prevented accidental slippage. Thirdly, it is a useful method in treating patients with giant IOFBs complicated with severe corneal opacity and laceration. The limitation of our method which is open-sky approach itself might threaten the healing of cornea incision and neovascularization.

4.3.2 Posterior Segment Intraocular Metallic Foreign Body Existence of 10 Years Causing Chronic Uveitis and Secondary Glaucoma

A 49-year-old man presented with a progressive blurred vision, pain, photophobia, and redness in the left eye for 10 years and worsened for 3 months. He had a history of penetrating injury in the left eye 10 years ago and was diagnosed traumatic cataract and IOFB. There was no information about the ophthalmic examination and ocular symptoms of the patient at that time. He underwent a successful cataract surgery and intraocular lens implantation 5 months after the injury. However, it was unknown whether the foreign body was removed or not. Three months ago, he returned with visual impairment and intraocular inflammation in the left eye, and topical antibiotics and medical treatment were given for photophobia, pain, and redness. However, the symptoms were not alleviated. On presentation, the visual acuity was light perception and IOP was 46 mmHg in the left eye. The left eye examination revealed chemosis, corneal edema, flare in the anterior chamber, and stale iris laceration. The fundus was not clear. Ocular ultrasonography demonstrated only a vitreous opacity in the left eye (Fig. 4.12a). Neither X-ray nor CT revealed an IOFB (Fig. 4.12b). Systemic and topical antibiotics as well as steroids were given, but no improvement was seen in vision and sign. Because of a clinical suspicion of an IOFB in posterior segment and secondary glaucoma, a 23-gauge vitrectomy combined with trabeculectomy was performed. A 2-mm long metallic foreign body was found at 6 o'clock of ora serrata and was removed from the sclerotomy site (Fig. 4.12c, d). The stale iris laceration induced by IOFB and iridectomy for trabeculectomy was seen clearly (Fig. 4.12d). Two months after the foreign body removal, the symptoms of uveitis and glaucoma disappeared. The final BCVA was 20/100 and IOP was 13 mmHg without intraocular inflammation (Fig. 4.12f). The visual field defect significantly appeared at the final follow-up (Fig. 4.12g).

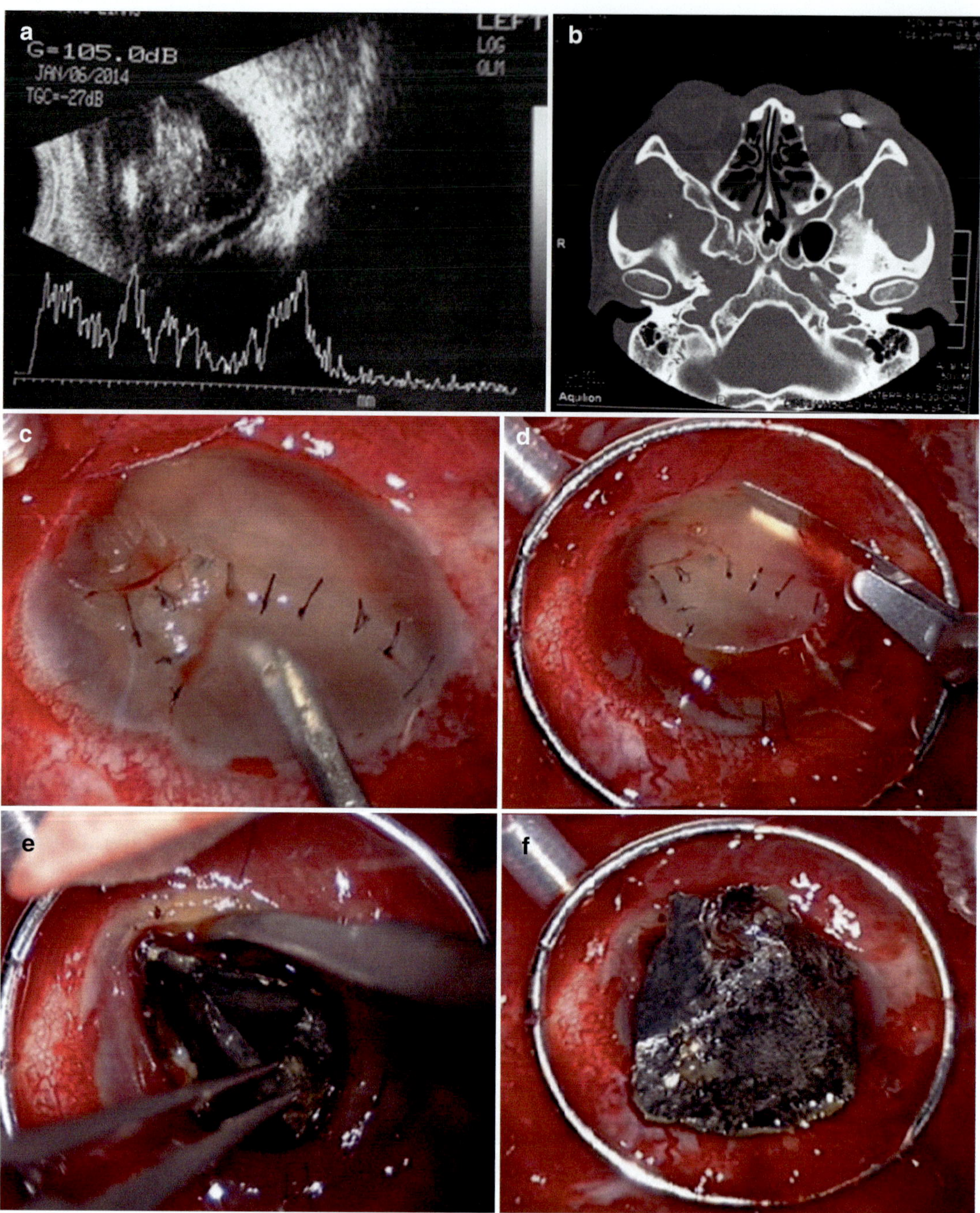

Fig. 4.12 (**a**) B-scan ultrasonography indicated a hyperechogenic shadowing that was concerning for a foreign body. (**b**) CT demonstrated a metallic IOFB in the vitreous cavity. (**c**) The irrigation-aspiration was performed for removing the exudates and hemorrhage in the anterior chamber. (**d**) The injured cornea was excised using a 7.25 mm trephine. (**e**, **f**) The foreign body was grasped with forceps and extracted through the open-sky corneal incision. It was an irregular-shaped and measured of 10 mm long, 7 mm wide, and 4 mm thickness foreign body

4.4 Current Consensuses on Intraocular Foreign Bodies

4.4.1 General Rules

As a general rule, a fresh IOFB should not be left in the eye after open-globe injury. However, if the IOFB is verifiable inert, and no signs of endophthalmitis was observed, early surgery should be considered carefully for its risk of potential complications may possibly bring more damage to the eye than the IOFB itself. In cases of posterior segment IOFBs, a decision of vitrectomy or not must be made in time: the more severe tissue damage is, the more indication of vitrectomy is given to remove the IOFB and prevent subsequent damage to the intraocular structure [12]. An invisible IOFB due to severe vitreous hemorrhage or inflammation is an absolute indication. Furthermore, decisions must be made depending on the condition of instruments, surgical timing, and preoperational prophylactic antibiotics [13].

4.4.2 Timing

The surgical plan should be well discussed once the IOFB has been accurately localized. Some IOFBs may be well tolerated, such as glass particles or alloys, and a decision of observation could be made in the first instance. This especially applies when the visual acuity remains fine. When an IOFB is decided not to be removed immediately, intravitreal antibiotics is wildly accepted and used as a prophylactic measurement against infectious endophthalmitis [14]. IOFBs in the posterior segment require to be carefully analyzed for the risks of endophthalmitis. Ophthalmologist should also consider the surgeon's experience and expertise, the equipment availability (at night versus in the daytime), the patient's general condition, and the legal environment [13].

4.4.3 Instruments and Management

Magnets Magnets are commonly employed for the majority of magnetic IOFBs (Fig. 4.13). Two types of magnets exist: internal rare earth magnets and external magnets. The iron content of the IOFB, location, and visibility within the globe determine which one to be used [15, 16]. External magnets are capable of generating great force but are bulky, restricted to use outside the eyes, and therefore, provide less control. Rare earth magnets are smaller, create a more unidirectional magnetic field, and are capable of fine control. They generated less force and are consequently restricted to intraocular use where they can be placed in close proximity to the IOFB. Their use in the posterior segment requires concurrent pars plana vitrectomy surgery. Inaccurate localization of an IOFB or incorrect use of magnets may cause numerous complications, including inadvertent traction on vitreous base and retina, or impaction of the IOFB into the lens [17]. The internal rare earth magnet requires the use of intraocular foreign body forceps for extraction since the type of magnet lacks the strength for trans-scleral IOFB delivery [18]. In most cases, even with external magnet, the IOFB is generally aided with forceps through the scleral as well [17].

Vitrectomy With the development of technology and instrument, vitrectomy still is the most widely used procedure in the management of posterior IOFBs, and intraocular forceps is also the most commonly used technique for IOFB removal [18]. Vitrectomy allows removal of any vitreous opacity and provides accesses to repair associated tissue damage. Vitrectomy instrumentation also provides a means of excising any IOFB-encapsulating fibrous tissue, and one may use gentle aspiration or intraocular foreign body forceps for grasping nonmagnetic posterior segment IOFB. In cases where the IOFB may be dropped, perfluorocarbon liquids may be utilized to dampen the impact and probably offer

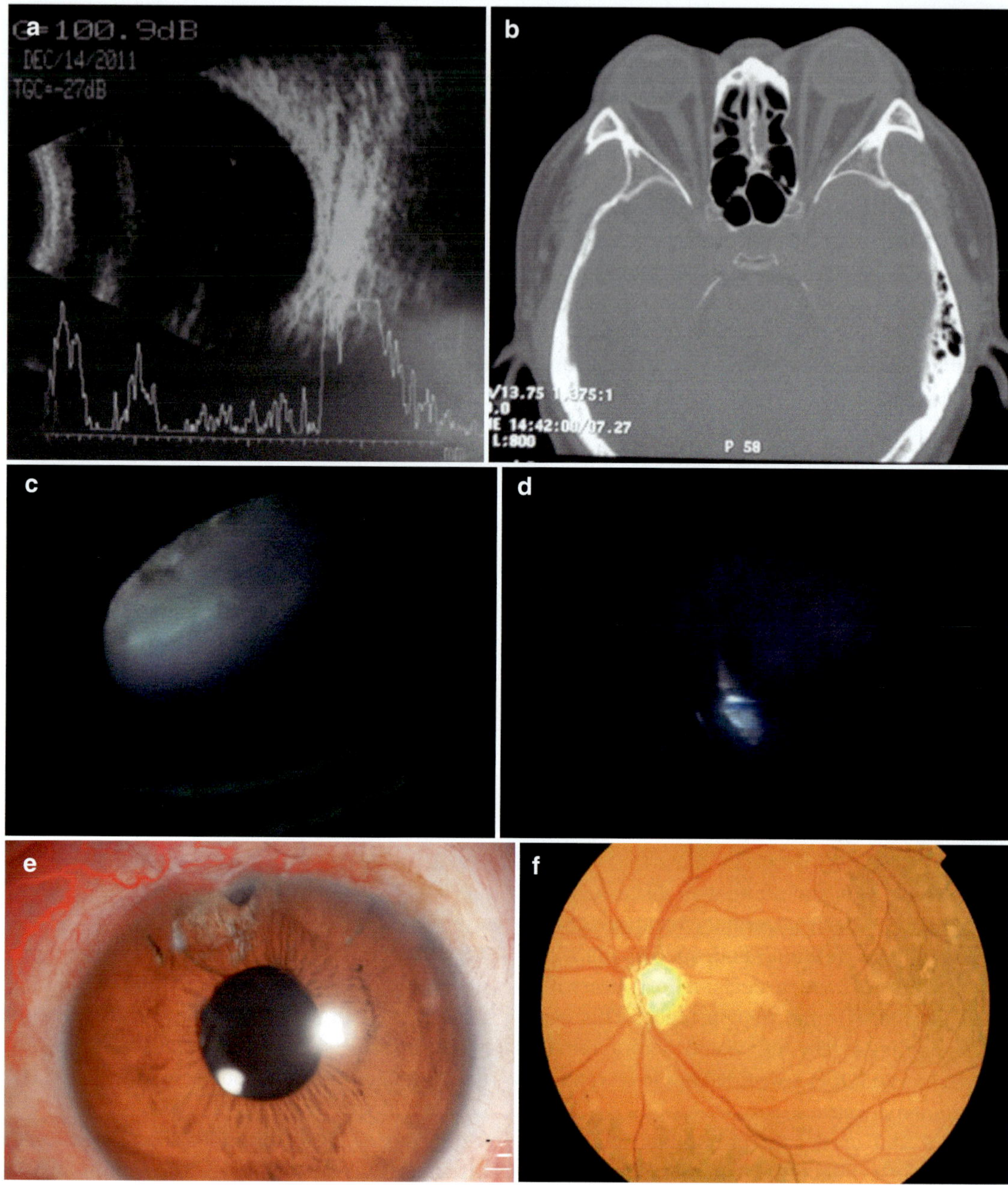

Fig. 4.13 (**a**–**g**) A 49-year-old man presented with a progressive blurred vision, pain, photophobia, and redness in the left eye for 10 years and worsened for 3 months. He had a history of penetrating injury in the left eye 10 years ago. Traumatic cataract surgery was performed successfully after initial ocular injury. Whether the IOFB was removed or not was unknown. (**a**) B-scan showed a vitreous opacity in the injured eye. (**b**) CT didn't reveal an IOFB. (**c**) A 2-mm long metallic foreign body was found at 6 o'clock of ora serrata in the surgery (*white arrow*). (**d**) The foreign body was grasped and extracted by an intraocular forceps (*white arrow*). (**e**) The stale iris laceration induced by IOFB and iridectomy for trabeculectomy can be seen clearly. (**f**) The optic nerve atrophy was revealed, and the ratio of C/D was 0.9. (**g**) Visual field defect appeared at the final follow-up

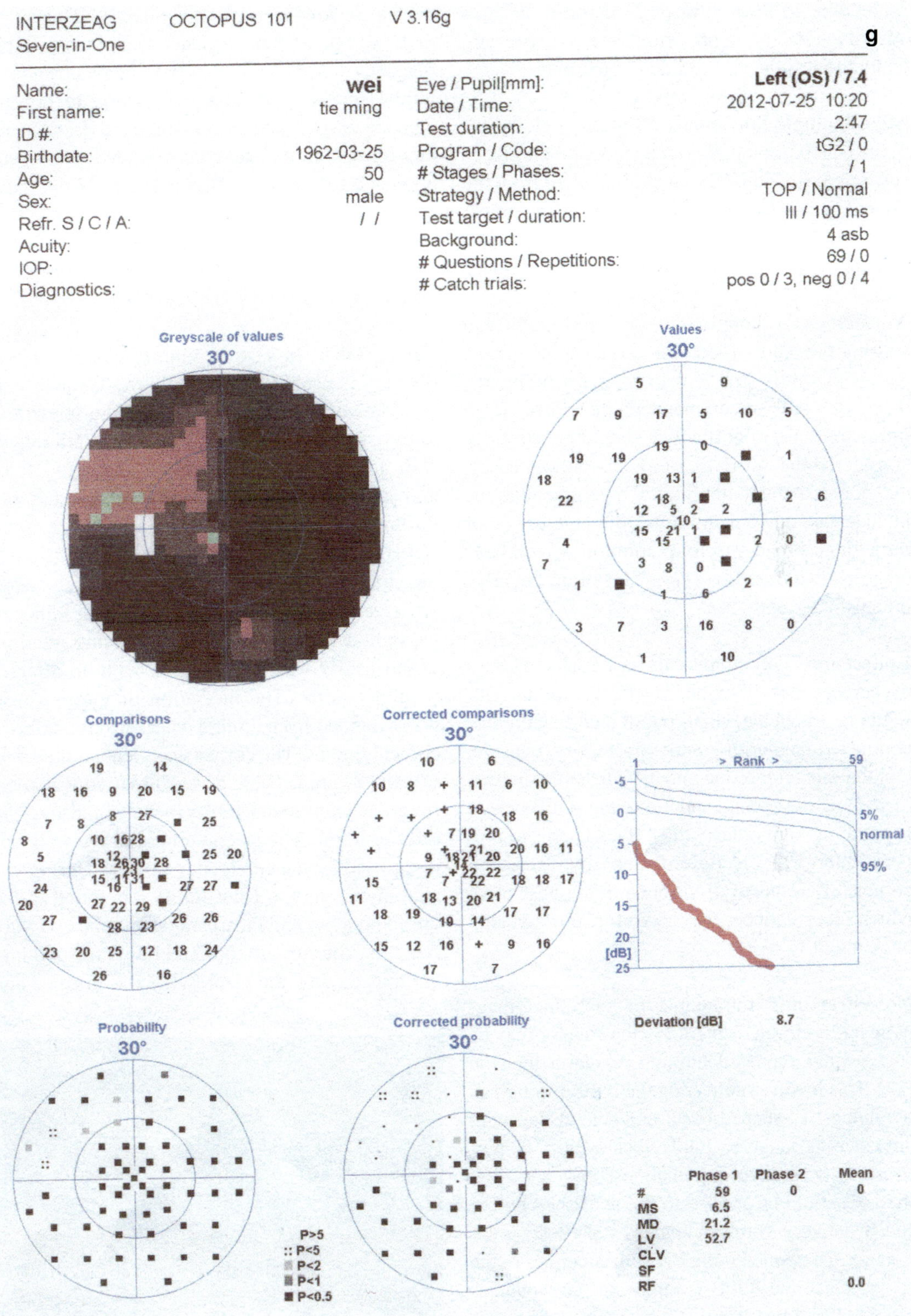

Fig. 4.13 (continued)

protection to the retina. Vitrectomy is also advantageous in the presence of lens disruption, endophthalmitis, and retinal detachment.

Microbiologic Specimens Microbiologic specimens can be obtained when endophthalmitis is suspected. Both the IOFBs and specimen from the injured eye should be cultured. Culture the object from which the foreign body arose, if possible. Culture the wound site, if it appears infected [19].

Antibiotics Although oral or intravenous use was not proved by literature to reduce the rate of endophthalmitis (6.8% with vs 7.2% without), they are still recommended generally [20]. Intravitreal use of antibiotics should be carefully considered in high-risk cases [21]. In those cases, the most recent antibiotic recommendations include vancomycin and ceftazidime, injection of intravitreal broad-spectrum antibiotics with coverage against *Bacillus* species and Gram-negative organisms.

Endoscope Vitrectomy can be limited in cases of corneal opacification, disorganized anterior segment, hyphema, small pupil, and opacified or contracted anterior and posterior capsule. Ophthalmic endoscope may be a feasible method in keeping the eyeball and removing IOFB before penetrating keratoplasty [22]. It also helps to prevent anterior PVR development by achieving completely removal of vitreous in the base area, which may reduce the need for prophylactic buckling [13].

No Vitrectomy Intraretinal or subretinal magnetic IOFBs located anterior to the equator may be successfully removed through a scleral incision [23]. This involves delivering the IOFB through an overlying "T"-shaped uveal and scleral flap with an external magnet. IOFB localization is performed by indirect ophthalmoscopy, and diathermy should be applied to the uveal bed before IOFB delivery. Surrounding laser photocoagulation may be applied if the IOFB incarcerates to the retina. Once the IOFB is removed, the wound is closed [17]. After removal, cryopexy to the retina and a scleral buckle should be typically applied to decrease vitreous traction indirectly. This technique can be used for patients with clearly visible magnetic IOFBs located in the vitreous or on the retinal surface without encapsulation to prevent damage of the lens and minimize the risk of cataract formation. It is not recommended to use such approach for large IOFB or when potential damage to the posterior segment is indicated. Very accurate localization of the IOFB is required, and vitrectomy may be inevitable if vitreous incarceration in the wound was suspected [13].

Giant IOFB In case of giant IOFB, pars plana delivery is usually hard to achieve. Limbal incision delivery may be recommended after vitrectomy, which helps to repair the retinal or choroidal damage, remove the disrupted lens, and move the IOFB into anterior chamber through the pupil. Figure 4.14 shows a giant IOFB removed out through a corneal limbus incision during vitrectomy.

A 22-year-old male was involved in an injury to his right eye from a metal stick. On presentation, visual acuity was hand motion with an afferent pupillary defer. The laceration of the eye wall was extended from 4 mm posterior to the inferior corneal limbus. The cornea was clear and the lens was not injured. There was mild vitreous hemorrhage. A giant metal IOFB incarcerated into the inferior retina. The laceration of the eye wall was just closed during emergency surgery. During vitrectomy surgery, a giant IOFB was found in the vitreous cavity and incarcerated into the eye wall. After the anterior vitreous and IOFB surrounding vitreous cutting, the giant IOFB was grasped and

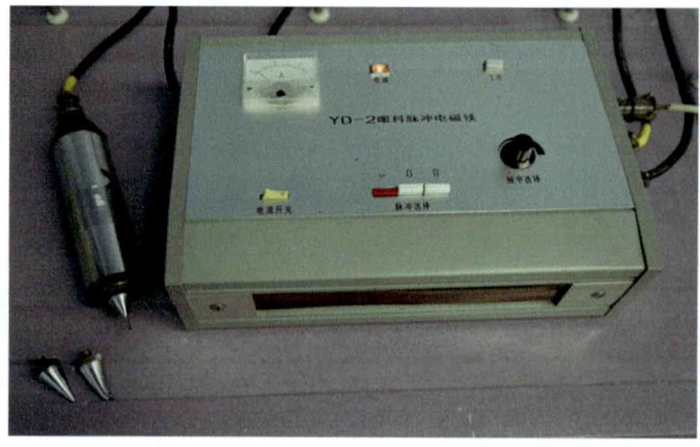

Fig. 4.14 Magnet used for magnetic IOFBs

moved to the anterior chamber, and then it was removed out through the corneal limbus incision. At the final follow-up, the patient's BCVA was 20/40, and there were no other serious complications such as glaucoma, proliferative vitreoretinopathy, retinal detachment, endophthalmitis, or ocular atrophy.

In this case there are several points of controversy on a huge IOFB removal:

1. Most of the surgeons choose to remove the posterior segment IOFB through enlarged sclerotomy, which carries a high risk of various intraoperative and postoperative complications, such as vitreous hemorrhage, hypotony, peripheral vitreous incarceration, and retinal detachment [24, 25].
2. Large foreign bodies can be removed through the sclerocorneal tunnel, but this may cause certain damage to the integrity of both anterior and posterior lens capsules [8, 26].
3. When an IOFB is too large to be delivered from pars plana, limbal incision delivery by transpupillary passage of the foreign body into anterior chamber should be considered. The huge IOFB through an enlarged limbal incision may induce obvious corneal astigmatism or incision-related complications [9].
4. Penetrating keratoplasty combined with extraction of giant IOFB is another appropriate approach in patients with severe opaque cornea. The pars plana vitrectomy combined with penetrating keratoplasty by using temporary keratoprosthesis has been commonly used in the injured eyes with a complex and multiple intraocular structure disorganization with favorable outcomes [27, 28]. Temporary keratoprosthesis allows a clear view for vitreoretinal surgery as well as creation of a clear visual axis.

Subretinal or Intraretinal IOFB Posterior segment IOFBs that are either obscured by opaque posterior media, composed of nonmagnetic material, too large for pars plana delivery, or embedded within the posterior retina, choroid, or sclera will require a vitrectomy to best ensure a minimally traumatic extraction [17]. To minimize the risk of iatrogenic retinal complications, encapsulated IOFBs should be fully freed before attempted removal [29, 30]. A retinotomy can be made for removing subretinal IOFBs, and a posterior hyaloidectomy can be performed in cases of intraretinal IOFBs. Sharp instruments (microvitrectomy blade, needle, scissors) can be adopted to adequately open the commonly strong capsule [13].

A 42-year-old male was involved in a hammering injury to his left eye with an IOFB. The visual acuity was hand motion, and an afferent pupillary defer was positive. There was a laceration evident that extended from 5 mm posterior to the temporal corneal limbus. The cornea was clear and the lens was not injured. There was moderate vitreous hemorrhage which blocked the view posteriorly.

During vitrectomy, a posterior segment metal foreign body was found embedded within the posterior retina just around macular area. After posterior vitreous detachment (PVD) was performed, we made a retinotomy at the IOFB area (Fig. 4.15a). The subretinal IOFB was completely freed and grasped by the IOFB forceps and was removed out from the sclerotomy site (Fig. 4.15b). The completely posterior hyaloidectomy, proliferative membrane peeling, air-fluid exchange, and laser photocoagulation were conducted then. One month later, the visual acuity was 20/200 with no vitreous hemorrhage, and the retina attached.

The highlights in managing subretinal or intraretinal IOFB include:

1. Subretinal or intraretinal IOFBs are usually obscured by opaque posterior media, thus imaging tests play a key role preoperatively.
2. For a subretinal or intraretinal IOFB, intraoperative retinal cautery is needed before retinotomy for alleviating retinal hemorrhage. Completely freeing the IOFB is the wise choice before it is removed for avoiding the tractional retinal detachment.
3. Completely posterior vitreous detachment and vitrectomy should be performed after IOFB removal for preventing postoperative PVR.

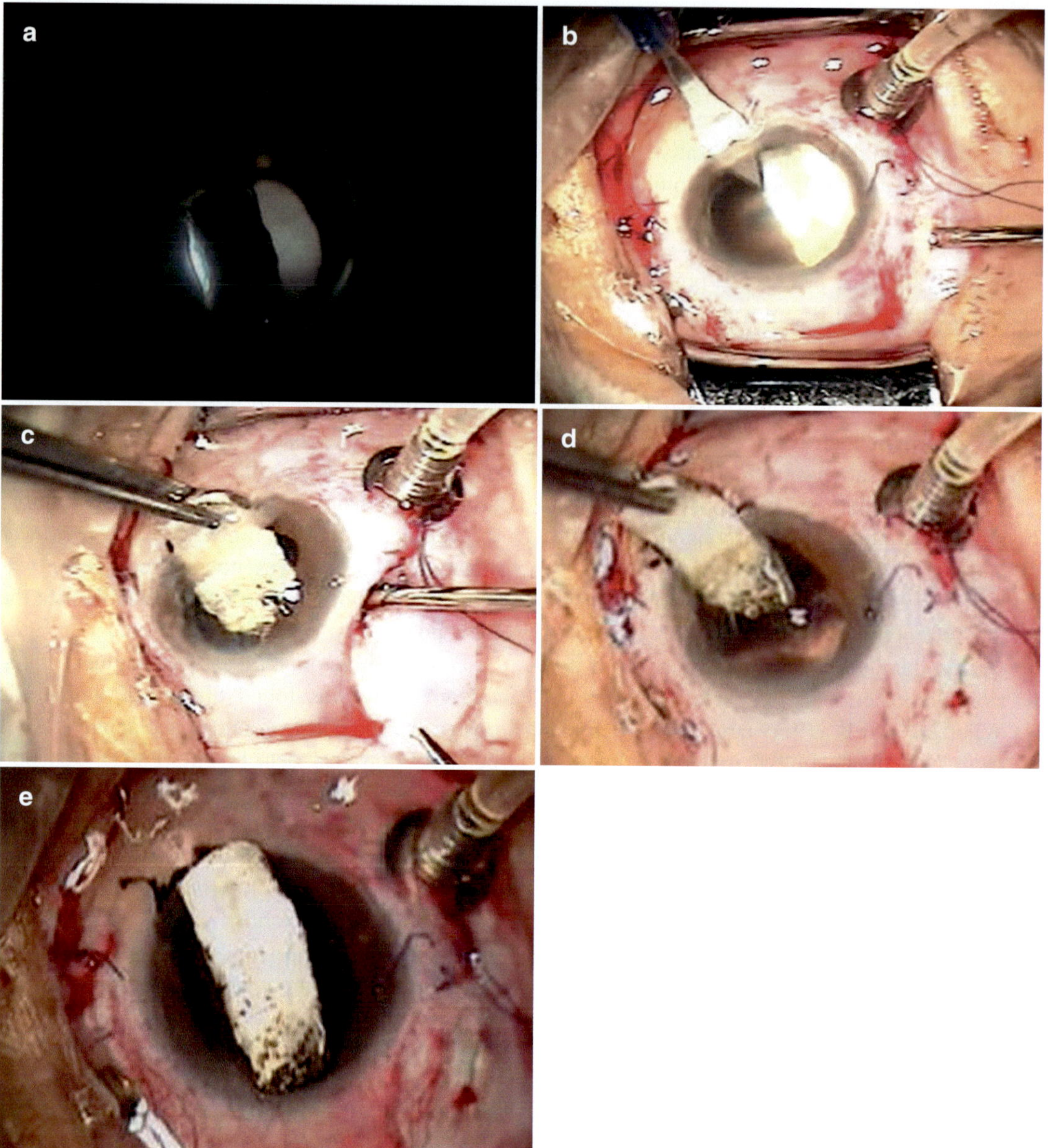

Fig. 4.15 (**a**) A giant IOFB was in the vitreous cavity and incarcerated into the eyewall. (**b**) A corneal limbus incision was made by 3.2-mm corneal blade at the opposite side to the foreign body forceps. (**c**) The foreign body was grasped and moved to the anterior chamber by a foreign body forceps and handed over to another forceps through the corneal limbus incision. (**d**) The foreign body was removed through the corneal limbus incision. (**e**) The full view of the giant IOFB

Suspicious Endophthalmitis Microbiologic specimens can be obtained when endophthalmitis is suspected. A pars plana vitrectomy appears beneficial for extraction of toxins from the eye, decreasing the infectious load, and possibly limiting the development of endophthalmitis.

Corneal Opacity Ophthalmic endoscope may be a feasible method if adequate visualization of posterior segment is prevented by intensive corneal opacity [31]. Temporary keratoprosthesis also offers a clear visual axis anteriorly and allows comprehensive reconstruction of the posterior segment [32].

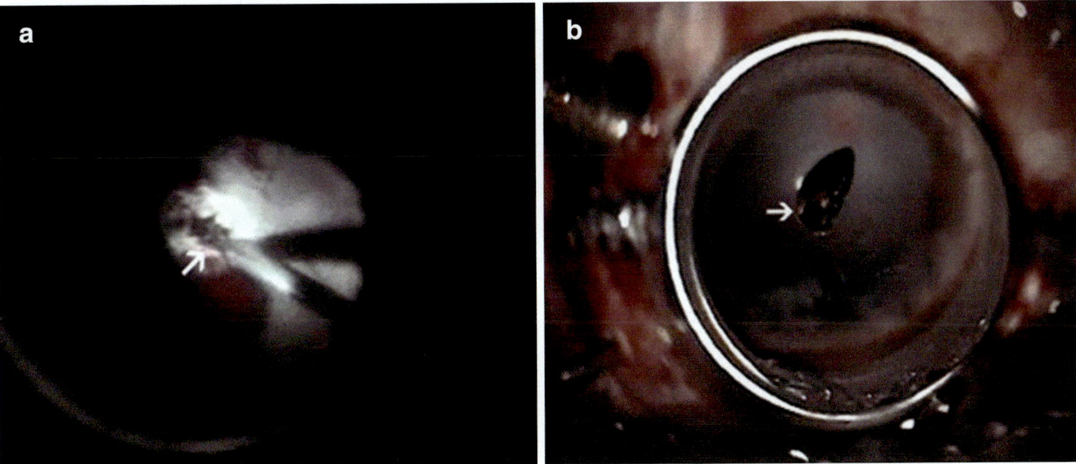

Fig. 4.16 (**a**) The intraretinal IOFB was isolated by MVR blade (*white arrow*). (**b**) The intraretinal IOFB was removed out of the eye through sclerotomy (*white arrow*)

Lens Injury In cases complicated with lens injury, primary intraocular lens (IOL) implantation is not usually recommended [33], especially with the presence of pars plana wound. Primary IOL implantation is available in some cases; however, the presence of IOL makes the secondary reconstruction more difficult [13]. In those eyes with intact posterior capsule, secondary implantation of a fixed posterior chamber IOL may be a better choice.

4.5 Current Controversies and Alternative Management for Intraocular Foreign Bodies

The controversy is always about balancing the benefits and risks. Doctors always make a decision to do what they believed benefits over risks.

4.5.1 Controversy 1: Timing of IOFB Removal (Recent Ocular Trauma with Fresh IOFB)

As a general rule, a fresh IOFB should be removed out of the eyeball as soon as possible. The main reason of such an early surgery is to reduce the risks of endophthalmitis and other toxicities induced by the IOFB, such as siderosis, chalcosis, or so [34]. In cases of IOFBs with high risk of infectious endophthalmitis, immediate surgery is usually indicated without doubt. Some studies also show that an IOFB removal within 24 h can reduce the risk of endophthalmitis significantly [35, 36]. However, some other studies showed that a delayed surgery for an IOFB with full evaluation and intravitreal antibiotic treatment might not increase the risk of endophthalmitis [37, 38], and no significant association was shown between the time of IOFB retain and poor visual outcome [39]. IOFBs need not be considered an absolute indication for immediate intervention [40]. Furthermore, if the IOFB is verifiable inert, and no signs of endophthalmitis was observed, early surgery should be considered carefully for its risk of potential complications may possibly bring more damage to the eye than the IOFB itself.

At the early stage of open-globe injury, media opacity and tight adhesion of posterior vitreous body often make the vitrectomy and the IOFB removal hard to perform, even for well-experienced surgeons. Complications may follow with an unsuccessful surgery such as PVR, recurred vitreous hemorrhage, glaucoma or hypotony, etc. Delayed surgery may make the vitreoretinal surgery less complex in the following ways: (1) Delayed surgery often provides a spontaneous separation of posterior hyaloid face from retina surface [26, 41]; (2) Media opacity caused by hyphema, corneal wound, or edema will recover in 14–21 days after injury [42]; (3) In cases of hemorrhagic choroidal detachment, delayed surgery will allow for liquefaction of the clot [43].

Many surgeons believed that early removal of the IOFB may benefit the patient and maybe decrease the risk of post-traumatic endophthalmitis. However, a delayed surgery with close observation and reasonable use of antibiotics may possibly prevent endophthalmitis as well and provide fewer complications from surgery which may benefit the patient even more.

An individual decision must be made regarding to the following risk factors:

- The risk of endophthalmitis (if high, remove the IOFB immediately and give intravitreal antibiotics; if low, move on to next risk factors)
- High risks:
  - Vegetable matter exposure and delay to initial management [4]
  - Lens injury [44]
  - Soil contamination/rural setting [45]
- The toxicity of IOFB (if high, remove the IOFB immediately; if low, move on to next risk factors)
- High risks:
  - Chemically or biochemically contaminated foreign bodies.
  - Organic foreign bodies.
  - Soil-contaminated foreign bodies.
  - IOFBs containing copper may cause chalcosis. It can lead to an acute inflammation and acute loss of vision and should be removed as soon as possible [46, 47].
- Factors may increase the difficulties of early surgery, such as media opacity, hemorrhagic choroidal detachment, etc.
- Is the surgeon well experienced and is the vitreoretinal surgical equipment available?

4.5.2 Controversy 2: A Retained Symptomless IOFB, Remove or Not? (An Accidentally Founded, Symptomless IOFB from a Previous Ocular Trauma)

A retained IOFB can be accidentally found during regular physical examination. Some of them are inert, symptomless, and can stay in the eyeball without causing any problems like intraocular lens. Some doctors believed that removing such an IOFB by surgery can cause unnecessary risks and costs to the patients [48]. Complications of the surgery may lead to decreased visual acuity and even ocular pain from elevated IOP. Close observation would be their choice.

However, on the other hand, some other doctors believed a retained IOFB may have a potential toxicity which may not be present at the time but if left in the eye may lead to a delayed reaction causing problems like uveitis, retinal breaks, and glaucoma [49]. In that scenario, a surgery to remove it as soon as possible may be a wiser choice. So here is the dilemma: how can we know if the retained, symptomless IOFB is going to harm the eye and should we remove it or not?

An individual decision must be made regarding to the following risk factors:

- The characteristics of the IOFB. The risk of chalcosis and siderosis development must be weighed against the risk of surgical intervention.
- Potential dysfunctions. Thorough ocular examinations should be performed, especially ERG and VEP, to rule out potential dysfunctions which cannot be easily noticed by neither the doctor nor patient.

4.5.3 Controversy 3: An Intraocular Eyelash Foreign Body, Remove or Not?

An intraocular eyelash can be caused by ocular trauma or intraocular surgery such as cataract surgery. Although the eye can tolerate the cilium for years, acute inflammation caused by an intraocular eyelash most commonly occurs within days or few months. Some doctors prefer observation, especially when no inflammation is present. Islam [48] reported a patient with an intraocular eyelash following phacoemulsification cataract surgery. During a 4-year follow-up, the patient has no symptom of decreased VA, pain, photophobia, or monocular diplopia and declined surgery to remove it, preferred annual review. Another patient reported by Chattopadhyay et al. [50] was not that lucky. The intraocular eyelash he got from an ocular trauma 3 days before caused him an acute anterior uveitis, and the doctor had to remove it immediately by surgery. This indicates that the decision to remove an intraocular eyelash remains controversial.

An individual decision must be made regarding to the following risk factors:

- The causation of intraocular eyelash. An intraocular eyelash caused by a sterile intraocular surgery may have a lower risk of causing inflammatory response than which caused by trauma.
- The structure of intraocular eyelash. The bacteria and allergens which may cause endophthalmitis or anterior uveitis when introduced into the eye are more often to be found on the root of an eyelash from the follicle. It is reasonable to believe that an intact intraocular eyelash may be more risky to the eye than a half eyelash without the root.

Clinical Pearls for Treatment

Before operation:

- IOFBs should be suspected in all open-globe injuries until proven otherwise.
- Computed tomography (CT) scan should be performed routinely for suspected IOFB, while MRI should be ordered very carefully unless the IOFB was proved non-magnetic and cannot be clearly seen on CT.
- The number, nature, toxicity, size, and localization of IOFBs should be fully evaluated before surgery.
- Bacterial culture and drug sensitivity test of conjunctival sac samples before using of antibiotics should never be forgotten.
- Endophthalmitis is the worst. All efforts to rule out endophthalmitis should be made, and antibiotics (locally and systemically) should be used in time to prevent from it.
- The patient should be well informed about the risks of IOFB and the surgery.

During operation:

- In general, IOFBs should be removed as early as possible. However, in some cases, a delayed surgery may benefit the patient even more than early removal. This remains controversial.
- Most IOFBs are extracted from a new opening unless the entrance wound is large.
- For an anterior chamber foreign body:
  - Make sure the anterior chamber is maintained with viscoelastic when removing the foreign body.
- For a lens foreign body:
  - If the lens is removed, IOL placement should be deferred when vitreoretinal damage is suspected or endophthalmitis is present or is at high risk of developing.
- For a posterior segment foreign body:
  - All vitreous surrounding the IOFB should be removed before embarking on removal.
  - If the IOFB is impacted in the retina, laser should be performed before moving the IOFB or inducing a posterior vitreous detachment (PVD).
  - Intraocular forceps should be opened only when sufficiently close to the foreign body to diminish the traction of vitreous body.

- The IOFB should be aligned to make the thinnest part be removed through the port site first.
- Safe and slow IOFB extraction, followed by inspection of the port site.

After operation:

- The removed IOFB should be safely preserved and showed to the patient.
- Antibiotics should be used continually to prevent from post-traumatic endophthalmitis.

References

1. Adesanya OO, Dawkins DM. Intraorbital wooden foreign body (IOFB): mimicking air on CT. Emerg Radiol. 2007;14:45–9.
2. Rubinstein A, Riddell CE, Kafil-Hussain N, et al. Self-inserted intraorbital foreign bodies. Ophthal Plast Reconstr Surg. 2005;21:156–7.
3. Pinto A, Brunese L, Daniele S, et al. Role of computed tomography in the assessment of intraorbital foreign bodies. Semin Ultrasound CT MR. 2012; 33:392–5.
4. Parke 3rd DW, Pathengay A, Flynn HW, et al. Risk factors for endophthalmitis and retinal detachment with retained intraocular foreign bodies. J Ophthalmol. 2012;758526.
5. Affeldt JC, Flynn HW, Forster RK, et al. Microbial endophthalmitis resulting from ocular trauma. Ophthalmology. 1987;94:407–13.
6. Ahmed Y, Schimel AM, Pathengay A, et al. Endophthalmitis following open-globe injuries. Eye. 2012;26:212–7.
7. Parke 3rd DW, Flynn Jr HW, Fisher YL. Management of intraocular foreign bodies: a clinical flight plan. Can J Ophthalmol. 2013;48:8–12.
8. Yeh S, Colyer MH, Weichel ED. Current trends in the management of intraocular foreign bodies. Curr Opin Ophthalmol. 2008;19:225–33.
9. Singh R, Bhalekar S, Dogra MR, Gupta A. 23-gauge vitrectomy with intraocular foreign body removal via the limbus: an alternative approach for select cases. Indian J Ophthalmol. 2014;62:707–10.
10. Huang Z, Chen L, Zeng Y, Lin C. Clinical features of perforating eye injuries complicated with intraocular foreign bodies located at the posterior global wall. Eye Sci. 2013;28:180–4.
11. Kunikata H, Uematsu M, Nakazawa T, et al. Successful removal of large intraocular foreign body by 25-gauge microincision vitrectomy surgery. J Ophthalmol. 2011;2011:940323.
12. Ryan SJ. Traction retinal detachment. XLIX Edward Jackson Memorial Lecture. Am J Ophthalmol. 1993;115:1–20.
13. Kuhn F, Mester V, Morris R Intraocular foreign bodies. In: Kuhn F, Pieramici DJ, Ocular trauma principles and practice. New York: Thieme; 2002.
14. Galloway NR, Amoaku WMK, Galloway PH, Browning AC. Common eye diseases and their management. 3rd ed. London: Springer; 2006.
15. Crock GW, Janakiraman P, Reddy P. Intraocular magnet of Parel. Br J Ophthalmol. 1986;70:879.
16. McCuen BW, Hickingbotham D. A new retractable micromagnet for intraocular foreign body removal. Arch Ophthalomol. 1989;107:1819.
17. Boyd S, Sternberg P, Recchia F. Modern management of ocular trauma. English Edition. Clayton: Jaypee-Highlights; 2009.
18. Parol JM, Machemer R. Diamond-coated all purpose foreign body forceps. Am J Ophthalmol. 1981;91:267.
19. Kunimoto DY, Kanitkar KD, Makar MS, Friedberg MA, Rapuano CJ. Wills eye manual: office and emergency room diagnosis & treatment of eye disease. 4th ed. Philadelphia: Lippincott Williams & Wilkins; 2004.
20. Thompson JT, Parver LM, Enger CL, Liggett PE, Mieler WF. Infectious endophthalmitis after penetrating injuries with retained intraocular foreign bodies. Ophthalmology. 1993;100:1468–74.
21. Mieler WF, Ellis MK, Williams DF, Han DP. Retained intraocular foreign bodies and endophthalmitis. Ophthalmology. 1990;97:1532–8.
22. Sabti KA, Raizada S. Endoscope-assisted pars plana vitrectomy in severe ocular trauma. Br J Ophthalmol. 2012;96:1399–403.
23. Joondeph BC, Flynn Jr HW. Management of subretinal foreign bodies with a cannulated extrusion needle. Am J Ophthalmol. 1990;110:250.
24. Chiquet C, Zech JC, Denis P, Adelinp P, Trepsat C. Intraocular foreign bodies. Factor influencing final visual outcome. Acta Ophthalmol Scand. 1999;77:321–5.
25. Wani VB, Al-Ajmi M, Thalib L, Azad RV, Abul M, Al-Ghanim M, Sabti K. Vitrectomy for posterior segment intraocular foreign bodies: visual results and prognostic factors. Retina. 2003;23:654–60.
26. Mittra R, Mieler W. Controversies in the management of open-globe injuries involving the posterior segment. Surv Ophthalmol. 1999;44:215–25.
27. Khouri AS, Vaccaro A, Zarbin MA, Chu DS. Clinical results with the use of a temporary keratoprosthesis in combined penetrating keratoplasty and vitreoretinal surgery. Eur J Ophthalmol. 2010;20:885–91.
28. Garcia-Valenzuela E, Blair NP, Shapiro MJ, Gieser JP, Resnick KI, Solomon MJ, Sugar J. Outcome of vitreoretinal surgery and penetrating keratoplasty using temporary keratoprosthesis. Retina. 1999;19:424–9.

29. Kuhn F, Kovacs B. Management of postequatorial magnetic intraretinal foreign bodies. Int Ophthalmol. 1989;13:321–5.
30. Slusher MM, Sarin LK, Federman JL. Management of intraretinal foreign bodies. Ophthalmology. 1982;89:369–73.
31. Norris JL, Cleasby GW. Intraocular foreign body removal by endoscopy. Ann Ophthalmol. 1982;14:371–2.
32. Kuhn F, Witherspoon CD, Morris R. Endoscopic surgery vs. temporary keratoprosthesis vitrectomy. Arch Ophthalmol. 1991;109:768.
33. Simddy W. Contact lenses for visual rehabilitation after corneal laceration repair. Ophthalmology. 1989;96:293.
34. Colucciello M. Posterior-segment IOFB treatment: timing and approach. Retin Physician. 2013;10:17–9.
35. Jonas JB, Budde WM. Early versus late removal of retained intraocular foreign bodies. Retina. 1999;19:193–7.
36. Lansing M, Glaser B, Liss H, et al. The effect of pars plana vitrectomy and transforming growth factor-beta 2 without epiretinal membrane peeling on full-thickness macular holes. Ophthalmology. 1993;100:868–72.
37. El-Asrar AM, Al-Amro SA, Khan NM, et al. Visual outcome and prognostic factors after vitrectomy for posterior segment foreign bodies. Eur J Ophthalmol. 2000;10:304–11.
38. Mester V, Kuhn F. Ferrous intraocular foreign bodies retained in the posterior segment: management options and results. Int Ophthalmol. 2000;22:355–62.
39. Wickham L, Xing W, Bunce C, et al. Outcomes of surgery for posterior segment intraocular foreign bodies-a retrospective review of 17 years of clinical experience. Graefes Arch Clin Exp Ophthalmol. 2006;244:1620–6.
40. Karel I, Diblik P. Management of posterior segment foreign bodies and longterm results. Eur J Ophthalmol. 1995;5:113–8.
41. Ahmadieh H, Soheilian M, Sajjadi H, et al. Vitrectomy in ocular trauma. Factors influencing final visual outcome. Retina. 1993;13:107–13.
42. Essex RW, Yi Q, Charles PG, et al. Post-traumatic endophthalmitis. Ophthalmology. 2004;111:2015–22.
43. Han DP, Mieler WF, Schwartz DM, et al. Management of traumatic hemorrhagic retinal detachment with pars plana vitrectomy. Arch Ophthalmol. 1990;108:1281–6.
44. Tompson W, Rubsamen P, Flynn H, et al. Endophthalmitis after penetrating trauma. Risk factors and visual acuity outcomes. Ophthalmology. 1995;102:1696–701.
45. Boldt H, Pulido J, Blodi C, et al. Rural endophthalmitis. Ophthalmology. 1989;101:332–41.
46. Cooling RJ, McLeod D, Blach RK, et al. Closed microsurgery in the management of intraocular foreign bodies. Trans Ophthalmol Soc UK. 1981;101:181–3.
47. Neubauer H. The Montgomery Lecture. Ocular metallosis. Trans Ophthalmol Soc UK. 1979;99:502–10.
48. Islam N, Dabbagh A. Inert intraocular eyelash foreign body following phacoemulsification cataract surgery. Acta Ophthalmol Scand. 2006;84:432–4.
49. Iqbal M. Consensus report. Retained intraocular foreign body. Pak J Ophthalmol. 2010;26:158–61.
50. Chattopadhyay SS, Dutta H, Kumar J, et al. Eyelash in anterior chamber, an unusual intraocular foreign body, following an indolent self sealing corneal rupture. Indian J Basic Appl Med Res. 2014;3:193–6.

Traumatic Endophthalmitis

5

Sengul Ozdek and Mehmet Cuneyt Ozmen

5.1 Introduction

Ocular trauma is one of the major causes of ocular morbidity and one of the leading causes of monocular vision loss. Over two million eye injuries are estimated to occur in the USA each year [1]. Post-traumatic infectious endophthalmitis is a particularly devastating complication of open-globe injury. Endophthalmitis is reported in 3.4 % of open-globe injuries [2]. Post-traumatic endophthalmitis should be analyzed separately because the pathogens that cause this condition are different from those in other types of endophthalmitis [3, 4]. To evaluate and establish a common language, a standardized classification of ocular trauma is a necessity, and the Birmingham Eye Trauma Terminology System satisfied the need being accepted by many authors [5–7].

Endophthalmitis might be infectious or noninfectious in ocular trauma.

A. *Noninfectious endophthalmitis*:
   1. Sterile uveitis
   2. Phacoanaphylactic endophthalmitis
   3. Sympathetic ophthalmia

   The pathogenesis of noninfectious endophthalmitis is through an immune complex-mediated granulomatous inflammation [8].

B. *Infectious endophthalmitis* can be caused by endogenous or exogenous sources [8, 9]. Each type of endophthalmitis is different in its microbiological profile, symptoms, and clinical course. Exogenous endophthalmitis can result from ocular surgery or trauma. All intraocular surgeries may be complicated by ocular infection. In most of the cases, infectious endophthalmitis involves an exogenous source rather than an endogenous one [9].

It is usually very difficult to separate infectious endophthalmitis and noninfectious endophthalmitis in penetrating trauma cases with lens rupture. It may start as noninfectious uveitis like phacoanaphylactic endophthalmitis caused by lens material; however, it may turn into infectious uveitis within hours. These entities will be discussed in detail.

5.2 Incidence and Epidemiology of Post-traumatic Endophthalmitis

Intraocular foreign body (IOFB) is an important risk factor for endophthalmitis after open-globe injury [8, 10, 11]. It is wise to assess data considering IOFB presence. Post-traumatic endophthalmitis constitutes approximately 25–30 % of all

S. Ozdek, MD (✉) • M.C. Ozmen, MD, FICO
Department of Ophthalmology, Gazi University
Medical School, Ankara, Turkey
e-mail: sozdek@gazi.edu.tr

H. Yan (ed.), *Mechanical Ocular Trauma*, DOI 10.1007/978-981-10-2150-3_5

Tip

Routine culture in all cases of open-globe injury is not cost-effective, as the finding of positive cultures at the time of injury does not predict outcome or change the management [19].

cases of infectious endophthalmitis [12, 13]. In the absence of IOFB, endophthalmitis rate goes down to 3.1–11.9% [13, 14]. With or without IOFB, the risk of post-traumatic endophthalmitis is higher in rural trauma associated with soil [15]. Cases of endophthalmitis can be classified as culture independent and culture positive. First group consists of all clinically diagnosed endophthalmitis regardless of culture data. Second group only consists of endophthalmitis with positive culture results [8]. One should also consider that the presence of positive cultures following open-globe injury does not mean that post-traumatic endophthalmitis will develop [16–19].

5.3 Signs, Symptoms, and Diagnosis

Post-traumatic endophthalmitis is a clinical diagnosis (Table 5.1). Diagnosing endophthalmitis immediately after an open-globe injury can be difficult because the inflammation and tissue disruption caused by the trauma might mask the signs of endophthalmitis [3, 8]. Pain and decreased visual acuity can be associated both with trauma and endophthalmitis. Pain from endophthalmitis might be differentiated from pain from trauma if the pain is disproportionate to the degree of injury. Other symptoms

Case 5.1

A 40-year-old male presented with typical infectious endophthalmitis 12 days after open-globe injury with a metal blade. Corneal perforation site had been sutured with 10/0 nylon on the day of trauma. Ocular pain started 7 days after the laceration. At the time of admission, eyelid edema, diffuse conjunctival hyperemia, severe anterior chamber inflammation, and hypopyon were present.

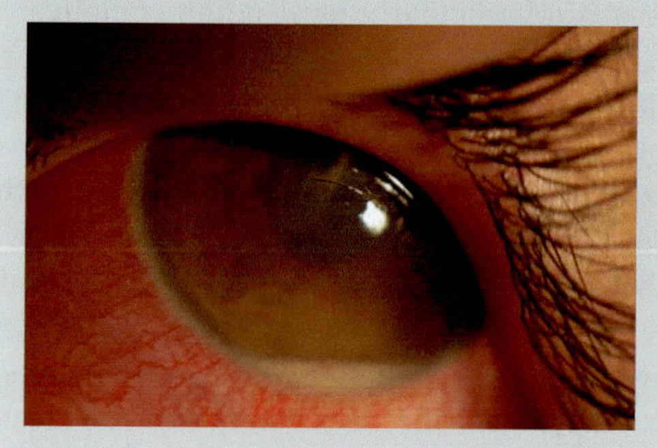

Table 5.1 Symptoms and signs of endophthalmitis after open-globe injury

Associated with trauma	Endophthalmitis before primary repair	Endophthalmitis after primary repair
Pain	Pain out of proportion to the degree of trauma	Increased pain
Visual loss	Visual loss worse than media opacities suggest	Further reduction in visual acuity
Eyelid edema	Eyelid edema	Eyelid edema
Intraocular tissue prolapse	Purulent exudation from the wound	Progressive inflammation
Corneal epithelial edema or erosion	Corneal ring infiltrate	Corneal ring infiltrate
No hypopyon (severe inflammation might be seen especially if the iris is involved)	Hypopyon	Hypopyon
Vitreous hemorrhage	Vitritis	Vitritis
No retinitis (retinal or subretinal hemorrhages might be present)	Retinitis	Retinitis
No periphlebitis	Periphlebitis	Periphlebitis

Modified from Ahmed et al. [20]

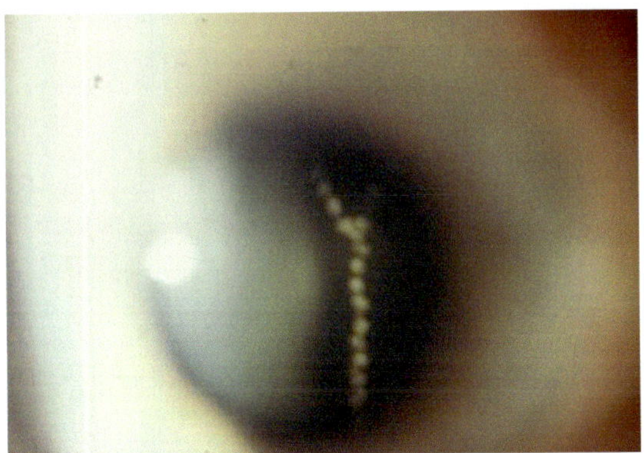

Fig. 5.1 Vitreous pearls in a fungal endophthalmitis patient

Case 5.2

A 38-year-old male was presented to our clinic with a 3-day-old trauma to the left eye. Visual acuity was hand motions. A self-sealing corneal perforation with negative Seidel test was seen. The typical picture of endophthalmitis was present (conjunctival hyperemia, severe anterior chamber inflammation, hypopyon, and vitritis) in addition to a ruptured lens capsule. Since we could schedule the surgery to the next day (which was the earliest possible time), we performed tap and inject procedure (intravitreal injection of vancomycin, ceftazidime, and dexamethasone) immediately (**a**). Computerized tomography of the patient showed intraocular metallic foreign body (**b**). B-scan ultrasound showed severe vitreous inflammation with attached retina and a hyperechoic foreign body with shadowing effect (**c**). Pars plana vitrectomy (PPV) was performed with lensectomy and IOFB removal on the next day (**d**). IOFB removal was done through anterior chamber. Mild retinitis and sub-ILM inflammatory debris were seen (**e**). Removal of ILM with the help of ILM-Blue was needed to clear the inflammatory debris (**f**). Fluid–air–silicone exchange was done at the end of surgery. There was no sign of endophthalmitis or inflammation 48 h after the surgery (**g**). Postoperative 1-month follow-up showed no sign of infection or inflammation, and best-corrected visual acuity was 0.6 with silicone oil in the eye (**h**).

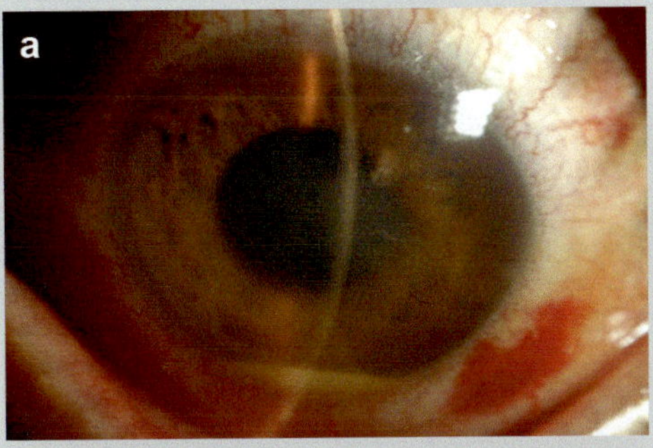

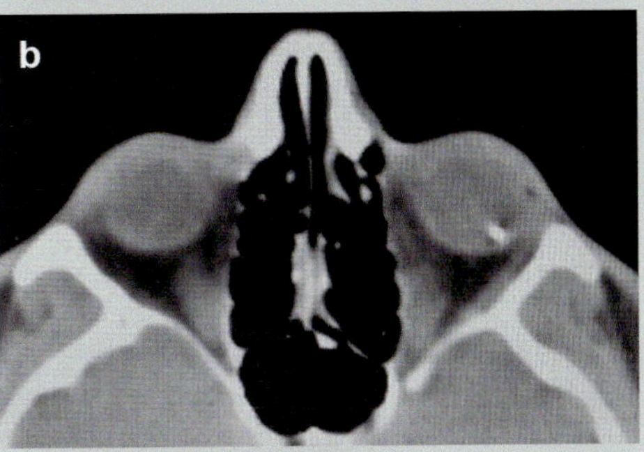

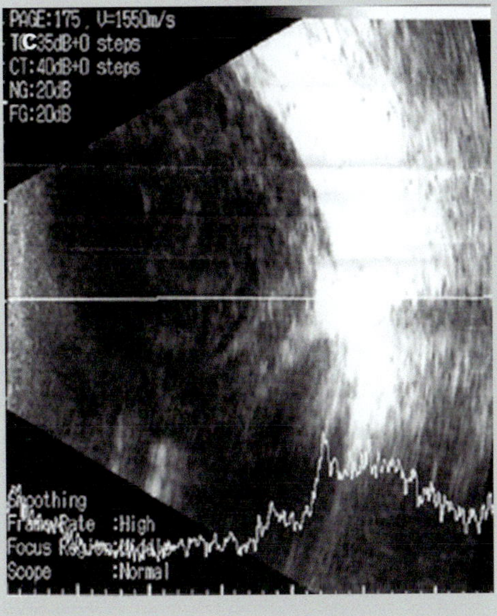

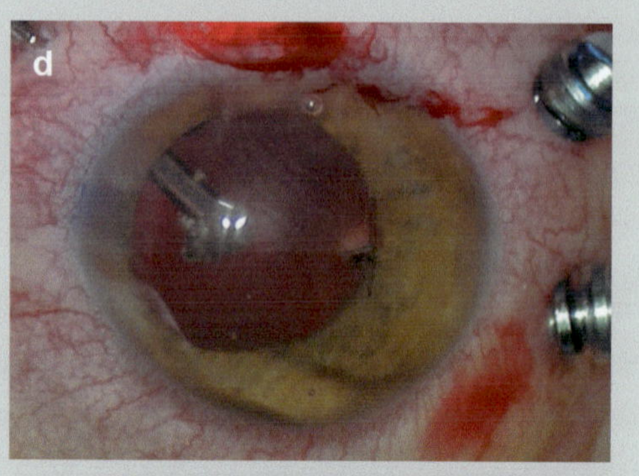

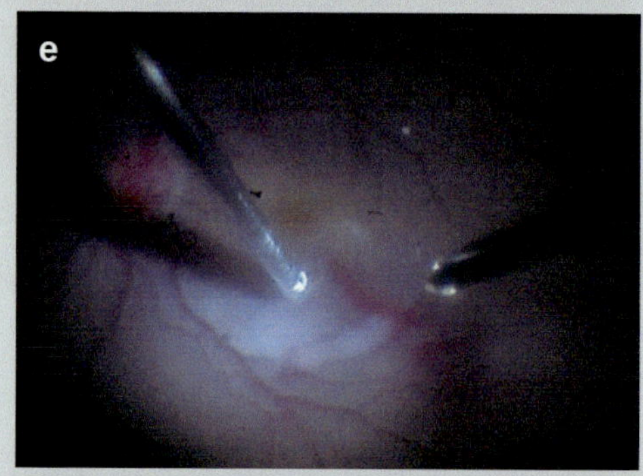

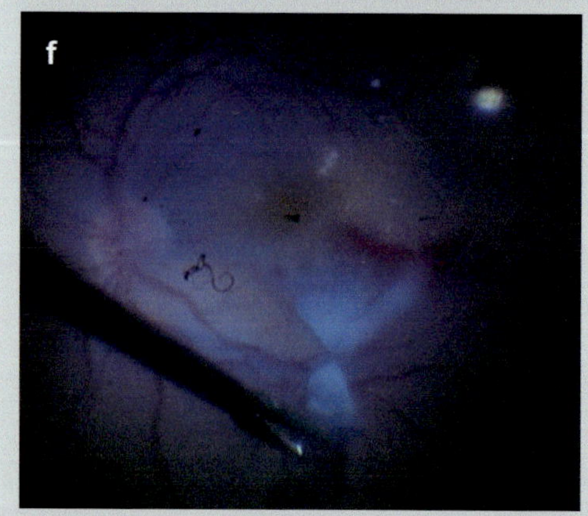

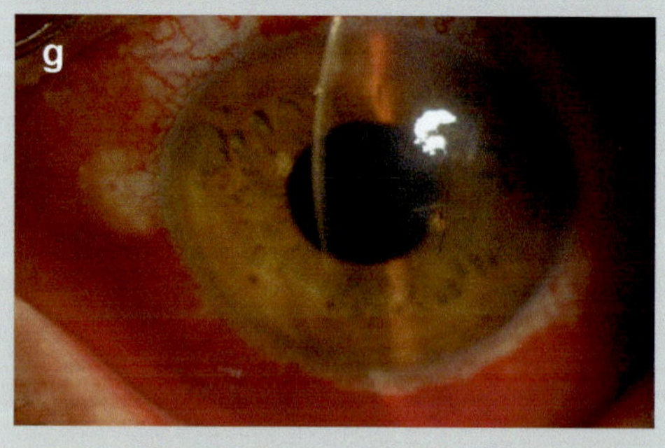

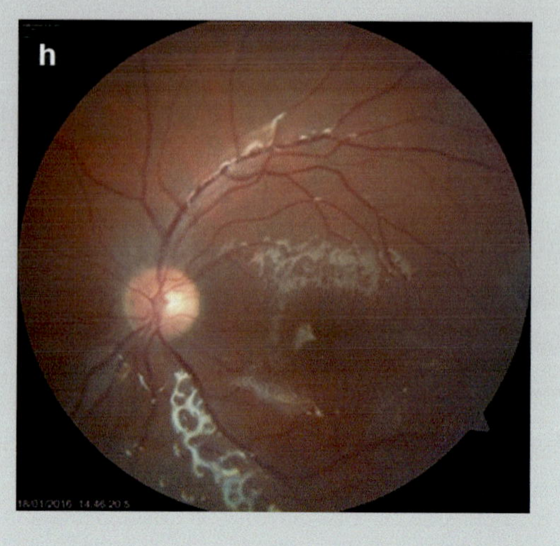

Tip

Pain from endophthalmitis might be differentiated from pain from trauma if the pain is disproportionate to the degree of injury. This may be an important clue before development of other typical signs of endophthalmitis like hypopyon.

might include photophobia, excess lacrimation, pain with eye movements, and ocular and periocular pain [2, 19, 21–23].

Clinical signs of infection include purulent discharge, edema of the eyelids, chemosis, corneal edema, hypopyon, and/or anterior chamber inflammation (pupillary membrane, posterior synechia), vitritis, and vitreous inflammation, and if the media opacity is mild to moderate, retinitis and periphlebitis can be seen (Cases 5.1 and 5.2a, d) [13, 19, 21, 22, 24].

A slowly progressing inflammation and vitreous pearls which are unresponsive to antibiotics should alert for fungal endophthalmitis (Fig. 5.1, Case 5.6) [2, 22]. In contrast to the intense pain in bacterial endophthalmitis, these patients have minimal discomfort. Clinicians should always consider endophthalmitis in eyes with a history of trauma regardless of the time of the injury since the onset of the symptoms might vary even after years from the trauma [8].

Symptoms of extreme pain supported by hypopyon and vitritis should indicate endophthalmitis until proven otherwise. If the symptoms and signs are subtle, diagnosis can be difficult. An increase in pain, inflammation, and vitritis and decrease in vision should support endophthalmitis. Patient should be monitored closely (even hourly) until the signs and symptoms improve or worsen to have a definite diagnosis [8]. If endophthalmitis is suspected, samples for cultures and stains should be obtained [16, 18, 22]. Cultures can be obtained from conjunctiva, wound, anterior chamber, or vitreous. Samples should be plated on blood and chocolate agar. Gram stain should also be performed [12, 16]. If fungal infection is suspected, Grocott's silver stain, periodic acid–Schiff stain, culture on Sabouraud's dextrose agar, or potassium hydroxide (KOH) preparation should be done [2, 25, 26]. Authors previously reported that DNA typing can rapidly and effectively detect fungal pathogens [27].

If infection progresses despite treatment, panophthalmitis should be suspected if signs of orbital inflammation are apparent, such as limited range of ocular movement, proptosis, increased eyelid edema, and erythema. During the assessment of post-traumatic endophthalmitis, all eyes should be evaluated for IOFB [18, 28]. In most of the cases because of corneal edema, anterior chamber inflammation, cataract, vitritis, and vitreous hemorrhage IOFB visualization may not be possible. Plain radiography, B-scan ultrasonography, and computerized tomography (CT) should be used to detect IOFB. CT sections should be less than 2 mm apart in order not to miss a small IOFB (Case 5.2b, c).

5.4 Risk Factors

There are many risk factors that are associated with increased risk of endophthalmitis after open-globe injury:

- The presence of IOFB
- Delayed primary wound repair
- Rural trauma
- Lens rupture and primary intraocular lens (IOL) implantation
- Large wound size
- Intraocular tissue prolapse
- Age (>50 years old and pediatric age)
- Male gender

5.4.1 IOFB

IOFB, as previously stated, increases the risk of post-traumatic endophthalmitis [10, 11, 13, 14, 29]. IOFB can affect visual prognosis in different ways: damaging the ocular structures physically (e.g., retinal tear), delivering the infectious organisms into the globe, and inducing damage with the chemical composition of IOFB (e.g., chalcosis, siderosis) [28]. The composition of the IOFB is important as studies have shown that nonmetallic IOFBs may have a higher risk of endophthalmitis [11, 14, 28, 30]. Copper IOFBs should be removed as soon as possible because they can rapidly cause sterile inflammation with hypopyon and retinal detachment, mimicking endophthalmitis. Ionization of copper leads to changes in neurosensory retina and if left untreated causes visual loss within hours [28, 31]. IOFBs with iron content can cause siderosis. Free iron ions interact with epithelial cells and cause cell death with visual loss [32]. Glass, plastic, and porcelain are inert materials which do not cause severe inflammation and are well tolerated in the eye [33]. All IOFBs (inert or non-inert) increase the risk of endophthalmitis [8] and should be removed as soon as possible.

High-velocity particles, caused by blast explosions and combat injuries, should have a special consideration as they have a less risk of endophthalmitis. High velocity of the explosion may increase the temperature of the foreign body leading to self-sterilization. In these cases visual outcomes are associated with the structural damage caused by the IOFB rather than with the timing of removal [28, 34].

In case of IOFB, early vitrectomy with IOFB removal is important as vitrectomy removes the source of microorganisms (IOFB), pathogens, and nutrients (vitreous) [18].

5.4.2 Delayed Primary Wound Repair

Delayed primary wound repair is a risk factor for post-traumatic endophthalmitis. The risk is higher if time between the trauma and repair is more than 24 h [11, 14, 35]. There is a fourfold increase in the infection rate when there was a delay of more than 24 h (Case 5.3) [10].

Case 5.3

A 35-year-old male with temporal corneal (zone I) penetrating injury who presented to another hospital *4 days after trauma for primary repair* was referred to us for endophthalmitis after primary repair. Visual acuity was hand motions with inflammatory fibrin membranes causing posterior synechia, hypopyon in the anterior chamber, and ruptured lens capsule. Retina could not be seen. An urgent vitrectomy was performed (**a**). Infusion was introduced through pars plana with anterior chamber maintainer being active during lensectomy. At this stage edematous corneal epithelium was scraped, and pupillary membranes together with lens particles were removed with vitrectomy probe (**b**). Visualization became better to see the severe vitreous inflammation (**c**). Following removal of vitreous membranes, retinitis and vasculitis signs were obvious (**d**). At this stage membranes at the ciliary body are seen and removed as much as possible with vitrectomy probe with the help of indentation (**e**). Surgery was completed with panretinal photocoagulation and silicone oil tamponade (**f**). Infection could be controlled and vision increased to counting finger (3 m) level, but significant hypotony developed despite of vigorous ciliary membrane removal during primary surgery. This hypotony led to migration of silicone oil into the anterior chamber, which had to be removed 2 months after the primary surgery. At the time of silicone oil removal, both vitreous cavity and anterior chamber were filled with an ophthalmic viscoelastic device, and pupilloplasty for temporal iris defect was also carried out (**g**). Postoperative fundus picture shows optic atrophy (**h**). Despite repeated injections of ophthalmic viscoelastic devices to anterior chamber and vitreous cavity 4–6 months apart, intraocular pressure was 2 mmHg.

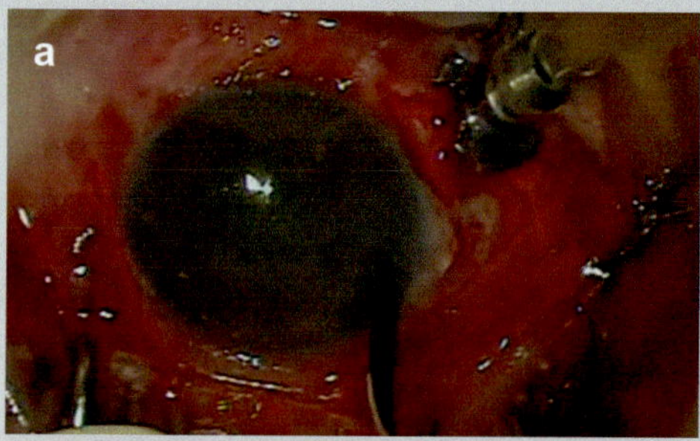

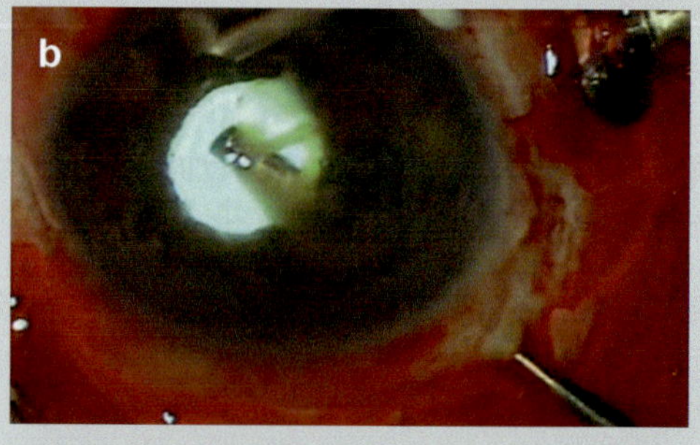

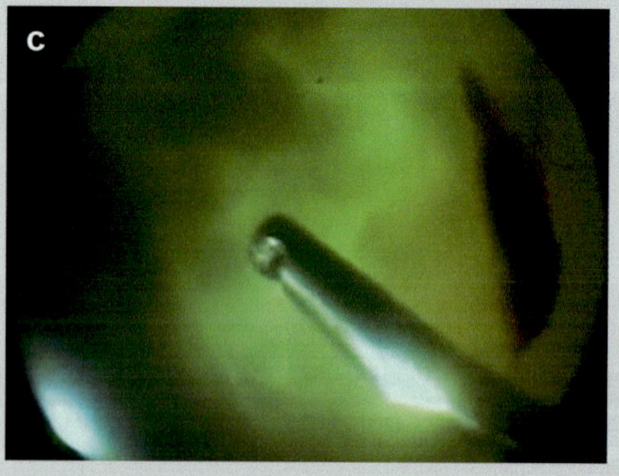

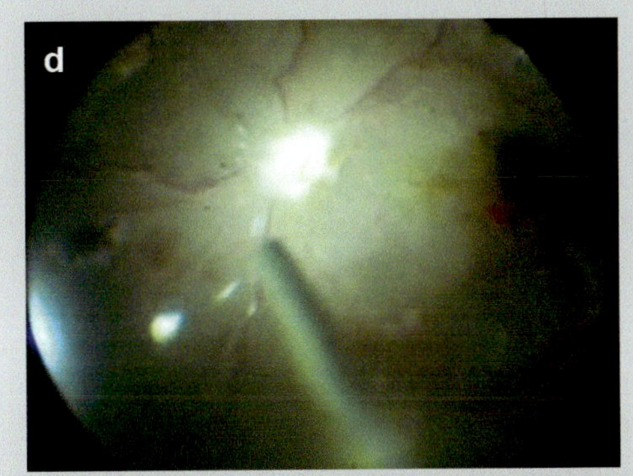

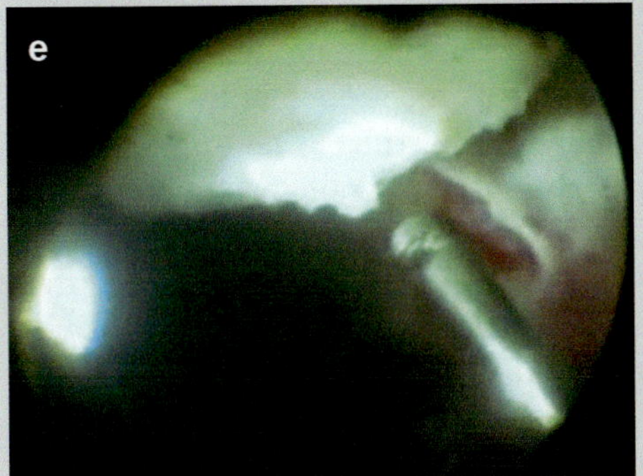

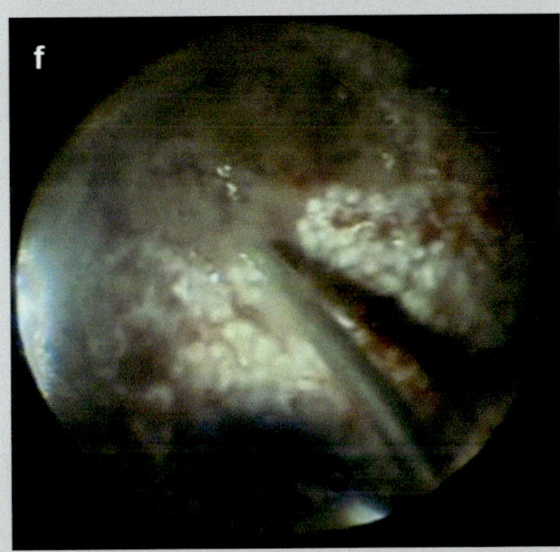

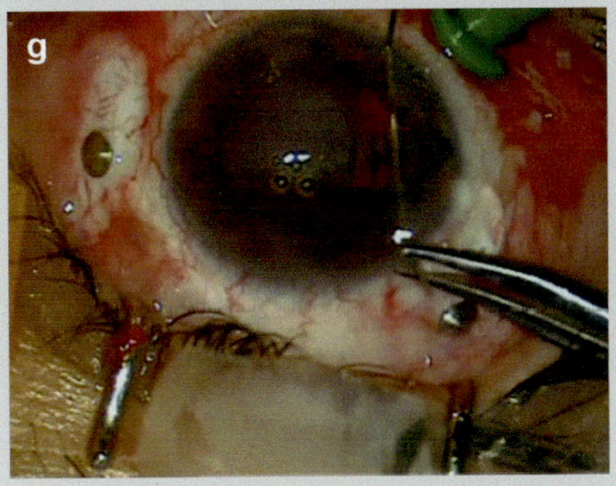

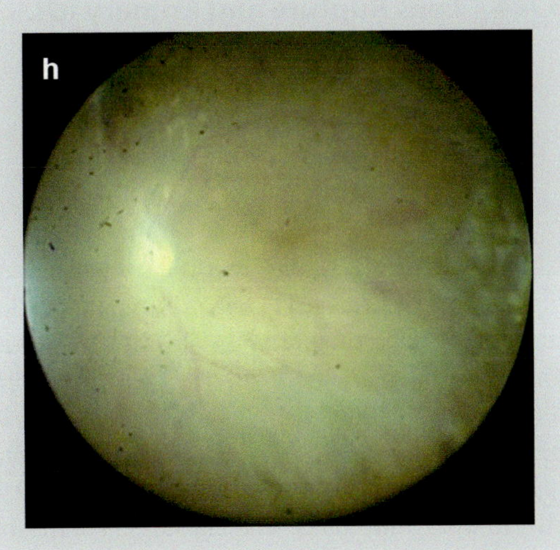

5.4.3 Trauma in Rural Settings

Trauma in rural settings increases the risk of endophthalmitis after open-globe eye injury. In these settings trauma frequently occurs after farm-related accidents with contaminated objects [11, 15, 36]. It has been reported that injuries with contaminated objects increase the risk of endophthalmitis [14]. The increased risk of endophthalmitis in open-globe injuries with organic matter may be because of increased microbial inoculum, more severe injury, and more resistant organisms [15]. Most common trauma which causes IOFB-related endophthalmitis in a rural setting is hammering metal on metal [15]. More than one organism is isolated in most of the endophthalmitis cases from rural areas. *Bacillus* species is the most common organisms in rural settings followed by *Staphylococcus epidermidis* and Gram-negative rods which will be discussed later [15]. Soil-contaminated injuries carry a high risk of infection with *Bacillus* species and *Clostridium* species, both of which are highly virulent.

Virulence of microorganisms which are causing the infection should also be considered. This issue will be discussed in Sect. 5.7.

5.4.4 Lens Rupture and Primary IOL Implantation Are Considered as Risk Factors for Endophthalmitis After Open-Globe Injury Separately

Although there are studies that did not show lens rupture as a risk factor [11, 35, 37], many studies suggest that lens rupture is a risk factor for post-traumatic endophthalmitis [8, 10, 14]. In two different studies, endophthalmitis rates were shown to be 12.8% [14] and 13.6% [10] in eyes with lens rupture and only 3.2% ($n=155$) [14] and 0.9% [10] in eyes with intact lens capsules. Thompson and colleagues hypothesized that lens rupture gives microorganisms direct access to vitreous cavity. The rupture of the lens capsule might also affect the aqueous humor dynamics and decrease the clearance of microorganisms from the anterior chamber [10]. Ruptured lens may also serve as nutrient and medium for the growth of organisms [10, 14].

Primary IOL implantation may be assessed as another risk factor for endophthalmitis following open-globe injury [8, 38]. IOL implantation is considered when there is lens rupture and there is adequate visualization for IOL calculation. Andreoli and colleagues reported in their study with 675 open-globe injuries that primary IOL placement is a risk factor for post-traumatic endophthalmitis [38]. In better words, it is not advised to implant an IOL during primary repair. It is safer to wait before implanting an IOL to allow the wound to heal and to allow the intraocular inflammation to subside. Additionally, during this period, clinician will be sure that there is no endophthalmitis following penetrating injury and a more accurate IOL measurement can be done after wound healing (Case 5.4).

5.4.5 Wound Size, Wound Site, and Wound Construction

Wound size, wound site, and wound construction are important for the visual prognosis and a risk factor for endophthalmitis. Lacerations (which are

Case 5.4

A 12-year-old boy presented elsewhere for a corneal penetrating injury with a small metallic foreign body also penetrating the lens and stopping at the back of the eye. Primary corneal wound repair had been done together with primary cataract surgery with implantation of IOL within 24 h in elsewhere. He came back with the full-blown picture of endophthalmitis 3 days after and referred to us at this stage for vitrectomy combined with penetrating keratoplasty. Vision was light perception and the cornea was very cloudy with a central laceration area; there was hypopyon and inflammatory membranes covering and blocking the pupillary area (**a**). An urgent vitrectomy was performed. After debridement of corneal epithelium, aqueous sample was taken for microbiologic examination. Following removal of inflammatory membranes from the anterior chamber, IOL could be recognized which was seen to be an ACIOL. Following pars plana entry, vitreous sample was obtained, and membranes covering back of the lens in the pupillary area were also removed which made the view more clear (**b**) so that we could proceed with vitrectomy without penetrating keratoplasty. After removal of central vitreous opacities, we could reach to a small metallic foreign body within opacities. We extracted the ACIOL to make the view more clear and to take the IOFB out through the same limbal incision (**c**). The retina could be visualized nicely after these maneuvers, and 360° peripheral laser was applied. There were edema and scars in the macular area but retina was attached (**d**). The eye was left with silicone oil and 1/3 dose of intravitreal vancomycin and ceftazidime at the very end of the procedure. Culture was negative for the case, but infection could be controlled very well after the surgery with the given intravitreal antibiotics and topical moxifloxacin + dexamethasone every hour for the first 5 days which was tapered later. Silicone oil was removed 3 months after and the best-corrected visual acuity remained 20/400 at the last follow-up because of the macular scar. Patient was left aphakic.

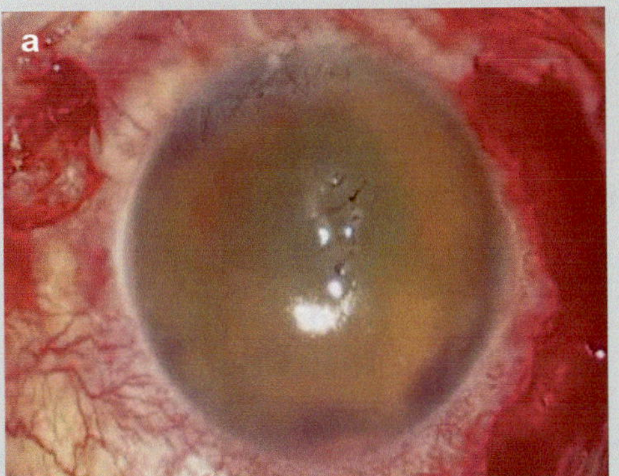

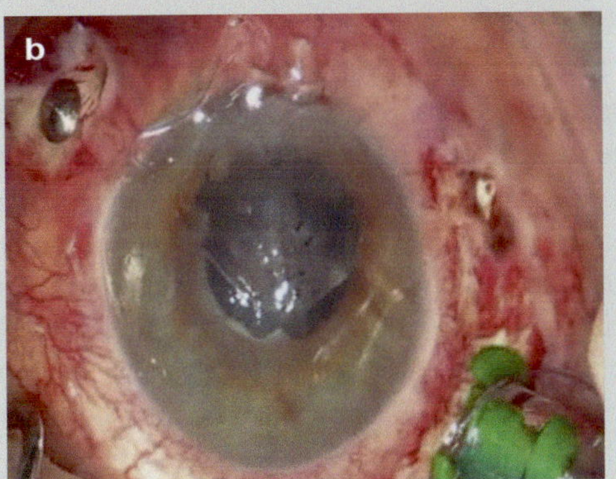

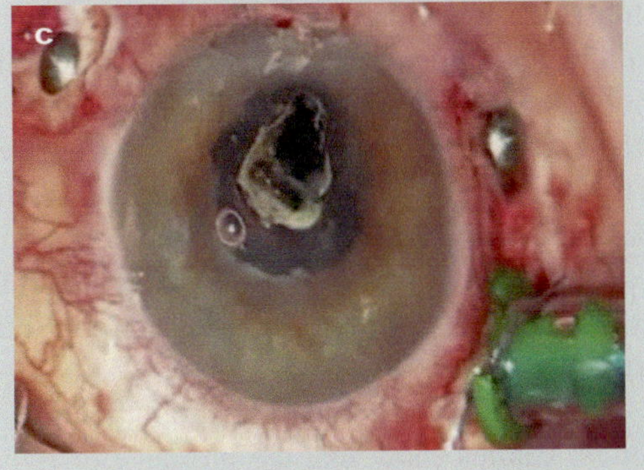

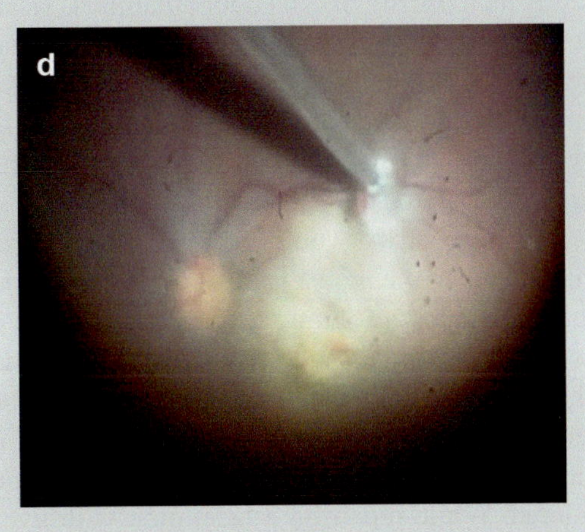

penetrating, perforating, or IOFB injuries) in general have a higher risk of endophthalmitis in open-globe injuries compared to ruptures [35]. It has been shown that more than 8 mm in wound size is a risk factor for post-traumatic endophthalmitis [39]. Although self-sealing of the wounds might be thought to be inferior to primary repair, it is shown to be equivalent to primary repair in protecting the integrity of wound construction [35].

Duch-Samper and colleagues reported in their retrospective study with 403 cases of penetrating eye injury that 2 % of corneal injuries developed endophthalmitis, whereas 7 % of posterior pole injures developed endophthalmitis ($p=0.03$) [40]. However in a more recent and larger study with 4968 eyes, Zhang and colleagues reported that 5 % of zone III injures had endophthalmitis in contrast to 14 % of zone I injuries ($p<0.001$) [35]. Zone III injuries might be protected against organisms by the overlying conjunctiva and Tenon's capsule.

5.4.6 Intraocular Tissue Prolapse

Intraocular tissue prolapse might expose intraocular contents to exogenous flora and organisms and was traditionally thought to be a risk factor for endophthalmitis after open-globe injury [37]. However Gupta [39] and Zhang [35] have reported that uveal or vitreous prolapse did not significantly increase the risk of endophthalmitis. Tissue prolapse may prevent invasion of exogenous organisms by plugging the wound, as well as it may facilitate invasion of exogenous organisms by forming a bridge through the wound. Further studies should be done to elucidate this issue.

During primary wound repair, prolapsed retina should never be excised. Prolapsed vitreous should be cut with sharp scissors, but excision of uveal tissue is not usually recommended because of the risk of significant hemorrhage [41]. Before removing the prolapsed uveal tissue, timing of the repair and wound hygiene should also be considered. While repairing a laceration with uveal tissue prolapse more than 24 h after the injury, the highly necrotic uveal tissue should be excised [41]. We also recommend removing the exposed prolapsed uveal tissue if the injury is of rural origin and there is significant debris on the surface of the exposed prolapsed tissue beyond the surgeon's ability to clean.

5.4.7 Age

Age was not shown to be an independent risk factor in multivariate analysis of the data for endophthalmitis after open-globe injury [14, 35]. However in two separate studies, Narang and Dehghani showed that low age (<15 years old) of the patients is associated with higher rate of endophthalmitis [42, 43]. Also Thompson and colleagues found from the 492 eyes with IOFB in the National Eye Trauma System Registry that post-traumatic endophthalmitis risk is increasing with age, especially in patients 50 years of age or older with delayed repair ($p=0.005$) [10]. We believe that children are at a higher risk for post-traumatic endophthalmitis development because of their low cooperation to examination which might delay the discovery of signs of endophthalmitis in coordination with their inability to tell the symptoms to their family which might delay the presentation to a clinician. We have three preverbal children who had accidental, self inflicted eye injury with injector needle, which was not noticed by the family and presented only after development of the signs of endophthalmitis. Since primary wound repair is delayed, it is not surprising that risk of endophthalmitis increases in these cases. Detailed information about pediatric post-traumatic endophthalmitis is discussed in Sect. 5.6.

5.4.8 Male Gender

Male gender to female ratio is reported up to 5.72:1 [35] which might be related to the gender ratio in open-globe injuries (up to 5.1:1 [44]). Zhang and colleagues found in univariate analysis that gender was not a significant factor associated with the development of endophthalmitis ($p=0.63$) [35]. Results of Essex and colleagues were similar and found that gender was not associated with post-traumatic endophthalmitis [14].

5.5 Pediatric Post-traumatic Endophthalmitis

Children tend to have a high rate of endophthalmitis after open-globe injuries (from 3.1 [45] to 54.2 % [43]). Clinical signs of endophthalmitis are similar to the ones in adults. However symptoms of post-traumatic endophthalmitis in children might be misleading. Depending on the age of the child, change in visual acuity and pain might be recognized late, and even if the symptoms are recognized early, the child might not bring them to the attention of an adult. This behavior may result in delayed recognition and delayed treatment of post-traumatic endophthalmitis in children (Cases 5.4 and 5.5) [43].

Causative agents of post-traumatic endophthalmitis in children are different than adults. In children *Streptococcus* species is the most common agent (25–55 %), followed by *Staphylococcus* (18 %) and *Bacillus* species (22 %) [46]. In adults it has been shown that *Staphylococcus epidermidis* and *Bacillus* are the most common organisms responsible for post-traumatic endophthalmitis [8, 21]. Fungal infection might also occur after organic matter injury [14].

Similar to post-traumatic endophthalmitis in adults, studies show that the presence of IOFB, rural setting, delayed primary repair of the injury (>24 h), injury with organic matter-contaminated objects, and involvement of lens capsule are risk

Case 5.5

An 11-year-old boy has presented to another clinic with a 2-day history of pencil-tip injury of the left eye. He mentioned about the injury 2 days after the trauma to his parents. When they arrived to the hospital, intravitreal cefazolin and gentamicin had been administered with a diagnosis of endophthalmitis. After 3 days of follow-up, hypopyon was still apparent and the patient was referred to us. It has been 5 days after the injury then. Visual acuity was hand motion. There was lead mark in the corneal entry site, corneal edema, and hypopyon (**a**). B-scan ultrasound showed some vitreous opacities (**b**). Urgent vitreous tap and intravitreal injection (vancomycin, ceftazidime, and dexamethasone) were performed. Samples were obtained from the vitreous as well as anterior chamber. Postoperative infection was controlled, but visual acuity remained hand motion because of the lens and vitreous opacities (**c**). One week after admission, a pars plana vitrectomy and lensectomy were performed. During lensectomy posterior lens capsule was defective, and inflammatory material was observed inside the lens capsule. Pars plana lensectomy was performed together with a complete vitrectomy. Posterior hyaloid was not removed because of its strong adhesions to the posterior pole. There was no retinitis. The case ended up with a fluid–air exchange. Two weeks postoperatively, there were no signs of infection (**d**, **e**). Visual acuity was 0.2 with a refraction of +13 D.

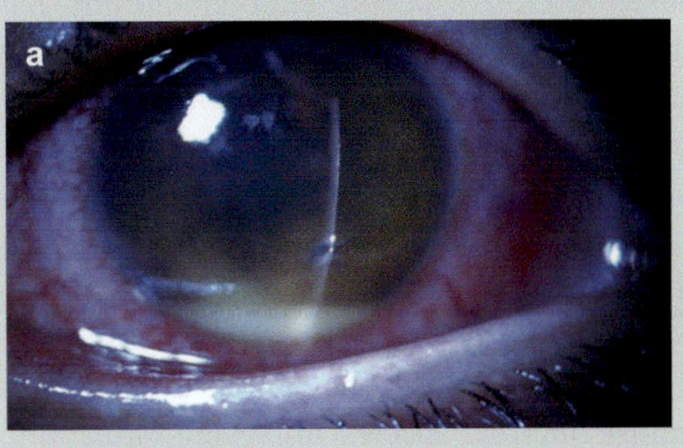

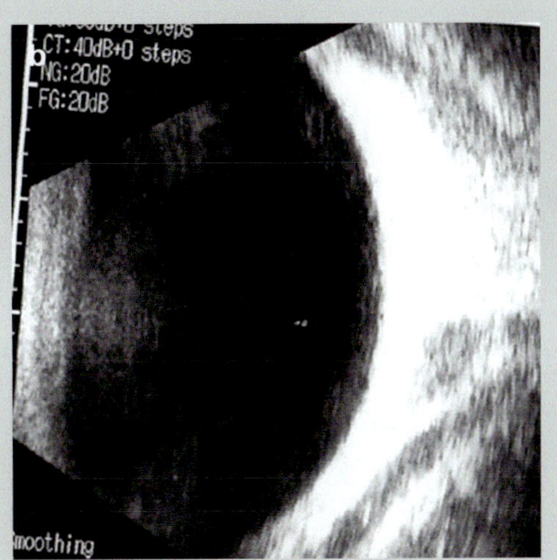

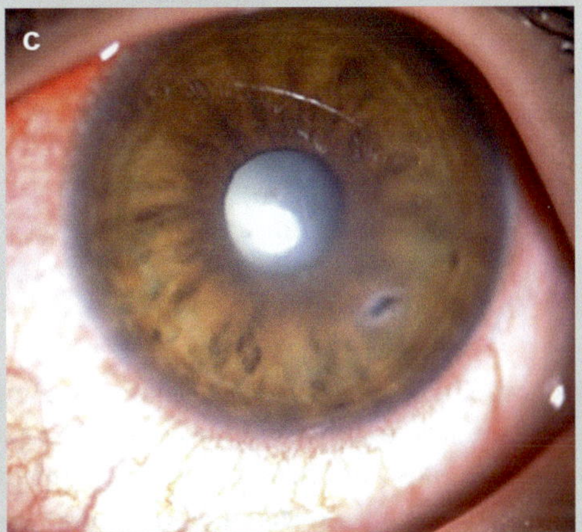

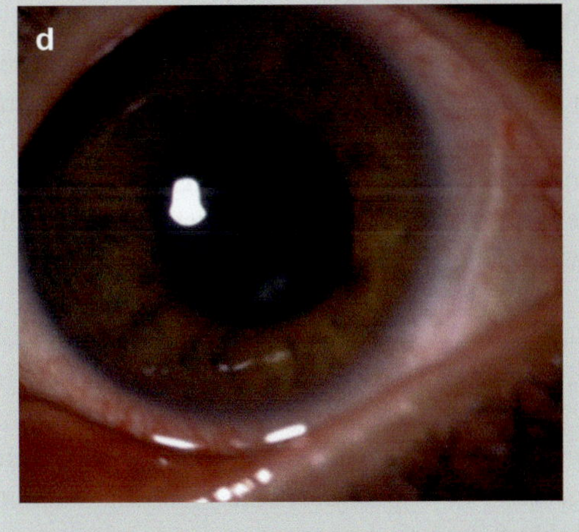

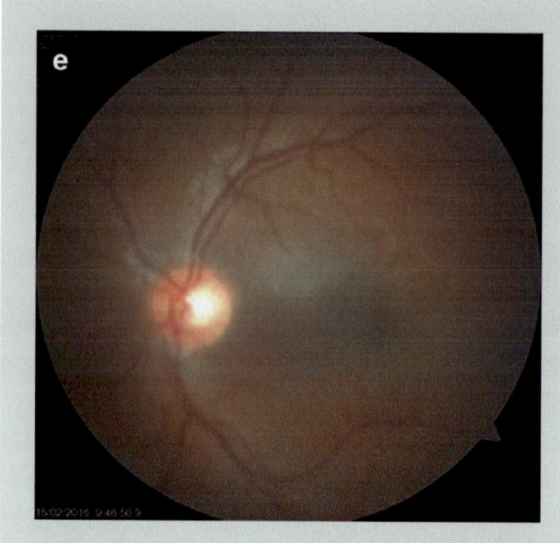

Tip

Prognosis of pediatric post-traumatic endophthalmitis is usually guarded both because of delayed recognition and treatment and amblyopia development.

factors [43, 47–50]. The rate of endophthalmitis in our pediatric trauma series was 12.1 % (22 of 182 eyes), most of them having late primary repair of the wound. Nineteen of them had vitrectomy, but only 15 % (three eyes) had a final VA of 20/200 or more [51].

A subset of pediatric patients who are 10 years or younger usually have a poor final visual acuity. Amblyopia plays an important role in this age group [21, 46]. However Narang and colleagues have showed that delayed primary repair is the major factor affecting visual prognosis [43].

5.6 Microbiology

Several organisms have been reported as causative agents in post-traumatic endophthalmitis (Table 5.2). It is important to keep in mind that without clinical signs of infection, positive culture results do not mean that endophthalmitis will develop [19]. Approximately 75 % of all post-traumatic culture-positive endophthalmitis cases are infected by Gram-positive organisms [21]. The most common organisms among Gram-positive species are *Staphylococcus epidermidis* and *Streptococcus* species which are part of the normal skin flora and thus contaminate open wounds regularly [52]. Post-traumatic endophthalmitis by *Staphylococcus* species tends to have a more favorable outcome compared to other organisms [53]. Intravitreal vancomycin and ceftazidime are treatment of choice in *Staphylococcus* and *Streptococcus* species [54]. Fourth-generation fluoroquinolones have excellent systemic penetration, and the MIC 90 for *Staphylococcus* and *Streptococcus* can be achieved with oral doses [55–57].

Table 5.2 Most common infectious agents in post-traumatic endophthalmitis [8, 20, 46, 52]

Bacteria	Fungi (8.3 %)
Gram positive (75 %)	*Candida*
Staphylococcus spp.	*Aspergillus*
Streptococcus spp.	*Paecilomyces*
Bacillus spp. (20 %)	*Fusarium*
Clostridium spp.	Dematacious fungi
Gram negative (10 %)	
Pseudomonas spp.	
Mixed infections (15.6 %)	

Tip

Culture positivity is defined by organism growth on two separate media, confluent growth on a single media and any growth in an anaerobic medium [8, 26, 34, 58].

When there is an IOFB or a penetrating trauma with soil contamination, the risk of *Bacillus* species endophthalmitis is higher (20 %) [20]. *Bacillus* species differs from other organisms in the onset and severity of the endophthalmitis they cause. *Bacillus* species endophthalmitis has a rapid onset (24 h) of severe pain and inflammation, chemosis, hypopyon, ring-shaped corneal infiltrate, and rapid progression to panophthalmitis. Its severity is likely caused by an enterotoxin-mediated reaction. *Bacillus cereus* infections tend to have a very high risk of causing no light perception [59]. Intravitreal vancomycin and intravenous vancomycin have a good coverage against *Bacillus* species. In severe cases amikacin can be added intravitreally. Fluoroquinolones also have a good coverage and can be added as an oral treatment [8, 20, 60].

Clostridium genus is a group of anaerobic spore-forming bacilli that are Gram positive [61]. Clinical signs of endophthalmitis associated with this pathogen include gas bubbles in the anterior chamber, amaurosis, and greenish-brown hypopyon [62, 63]. This organism is highly virulent and can cause endophthalmitis within 24 h with rapid progression and causing panophthalmitis [8, 63]. Visual outcome in most cases of *Clostridium* endophthalmitis is very poor generally resulting in no light perception [8, 61, 63]. Intravitreal vancomycin and ceftazidime can be used to treat *Clostridium* endophthalmitis following open-globe injury [64].

Gram-negative organisms are the cause of post-traumatic endophthalmitis less than Gram-positive organisms. They are reported to be the causative agent from 0 to 33 % of cases with post-traumatic endophthalmitis [52, 65, 66]. Although they are a rare cause of post-traumatic endophthalmitis, they are usually virulent, and the prognosis is poor. *Pseudomonas* is the most commonly isolated organism in this group. It has multiple drug resistance, and it is recommended to treat *Pseudomonas* with combination therapy. Tobramycin–piperacillin and tobramycin–ceftazidime are popular combinations. Fluoroquinolones also cover *Pseudomonas*, and ciprofloxacin, which is a third-generation fluoroquinolone, has the best coverage. Organisms that can cause fulminant endophthalmitis include *Bacillus*, *Pseudomonas*, and *Clostridium* species [67].

Polymicrobial infection is more frequent in endophthalmitis following open-globe injuries compared to other types of endophthalmitis (15.6 % [52]).

Fungi are less common than bacteria in post-traumatic endophthalmitis. The incidence of fungal agents is reported to be between 0 and 15.4 % [13, 26, 68]. The most common fungus causing post-traumatic endophthalmitis is *Candida* [23], but molds such as *Aspergillus* species, *Paecilomyces* species, *Fusarium* species, and dematacious fungi have also been reported [20, 69].

Differentiating between fungus and bacteria is important as their treatments are different. Late onset (1–5 weeks) of symptoms with a fairly asymptomatic external eye exam, slowly progressive intraocular inflammation, and/or the presence of vitreous inflammation (vitreous snow balls/vitreous pearls) might be suggestive of fungal infection [2, 70, 71] (Fig. 5.1, Case 5.6).

Case 5.6

A 36-year-old female patient has been referred to our clinic with a history of a traffic accident with penetrating eye injury 3 months ago. From the previous reports, we learned that phacoemulsification with intraocular lens implantation was performed after primary wound repair in another clinic. Three separate pars plana vitrectomy surgeries with silicone oil had been done after intravitreal antibiotic injections were assessed insufficient. IOL was removed at the latest surgery. Only the first culture yielded *Streptococcus* species. Three of the later cultures revealed no organisms. Cultures for fungi had not been performed. Upon admittance to our clinic, there was central keratitis, severe anterior chamber inflammation. We got samples from the anterior chamber and cornea for fungi as soon as we admitted the patient. Cultures yielded *Aspergillus terreus* with a susceptibility to amphotericin B and voriconazole. Although we have started empirically, intravitreal and intracameral voriconazole treatment phthisis bulbi was inevitable. This case demonstrates the importance of differentiating fungal endophthalmitis and its severe complications if diagnosed late.

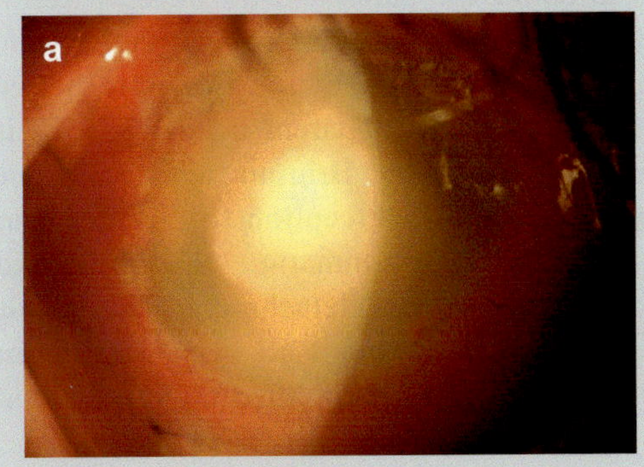

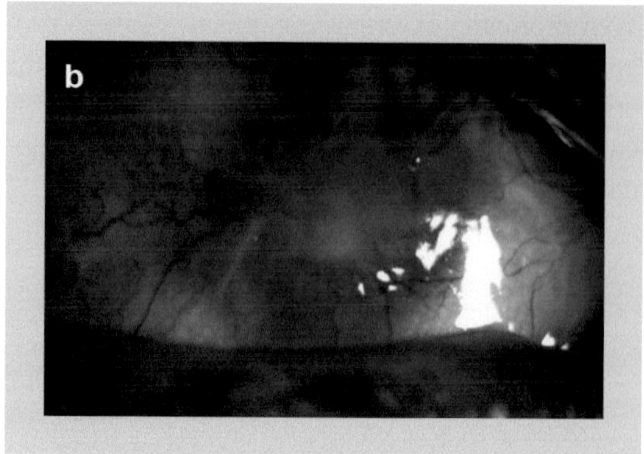

5.7 Prognosis

Visual prognosis in eyes with endophthalmitis secondary to trauma is poor. The visual prognosis is affected by the endophthalmitis as well as trauma itself [14, 35]. The effect of endophthalmitis on visual prognosis in an open-globe injury is described in the ocular trauma score (OTS) which can provide a probability estimate of the visual outcome 6 months after the injury [8, 72]. OTS calculates the probability considering many variables. Patients presenting visual acuity, the presence of rupture, perforating injury, retinal detachment, and afferent pupillary defect are factors effecting final visual outcome [72].

The status of the retina plays an important role in the final visual acuity. Retinal detachment and retinal breaks with post-traumatic endophthalmitis on presentation usually has a very poor visual prognosis [13]. Also the risk of retinal detachment after vitrectomy for endophthalmitis is higher [73]. Visual prognosis is better for patients who develop retinal detachment after successful vitrectomy for post-traumatic endophthalmitis than if the retinal detachment is apparent concurrently with the infection [74]. Brinton and colleagues reported no light perception to 20/200 visual acuity in post-traumatic endophthalmitis patients with retinal detachment [13]. Affeldt and colleagues reported all eyes with retinal detachment with endophthalmitis developed phthisis bulbi [74].

Virulence of the organisms should also be considered which has been discussed previously (Sect. 5.6). *Bacillus* species, *Clostridium* species, and Gram-negative organisms (e.g., *Pseudomonas*) are highly virulent and cause rapid onset of endophthalmitis (within 24 h) and visual acuity as low as no light perception can occur [3, 52, 62–64, 68].

5.8 Prophylaxis

Despite extensive literature on open-globe injuries and outcomes, currently there are no randomized controlled studies to establish the best prophylactic antibiotic regimen, and there is no standard protocol. Systemic antibiotics used simultaneously with topical antibiotics have been considered standard of care by many clinicians [75].

5.8.1 Systemic Prophylaxis

It is suggested that systemic antibiotic penetrance to the eye after ocular trauma is higher because of the disruption of the blood–retinal barrier. As a result oral and intravenous antibiotic administration is a rational option [76]. Vitreous penetrance with oral antibiotic administration has mostly been tested for fluoroquinolones.

Fiscella and colleagues studied the vitreous penetration of levofloxacin in 45 patients undergoing vitrectomy who had two doses of 500 mg orally administered levofloxacin 12 h apart. MIC90 concentrations were achieved for *S. epidermidis*, *S. aureus*, *Staphylococcus pneumonia*, *Bacillus cereus*, and some Gram-negative organisms but not for *Pseudomonas* or *Enterococcus* [77]. In a similar study, Herbert and colleagues concluded that more than one dose of levofloxacin is needed to achieve adequate vitreous concentrations [78]. Hariprasad and colleagues studied vitreous penetration of two doses of 400 mg moxifloxacin administered orally 12 h apart and showed that the drug achieved MIC90 doses for most common pathogens except for *Pseudomonas* [57]. The MIC90 values used in these studies vary which illustrate the subjectivity in these studies. MIC90 will vary geographically for each organism and will rise over time as resistance becomes more widespread [75, 78].

There are no studies that use oral antibiotics for endophthalmitis prophylaxis as a standard of care and report infection outcomes. But in a study with 69 eyes with open-globe injury, Woodcock and colleagues found that endophthalmitis developed only in patients who did not receive antibiotic prophylaxis and noted that majority of cases who received prophylaxis received oral ciprofloxacin [79]. And they recommended ciprofloxacin 750 mg twice daily for 1 week for prophylaxis but also added that patients with high-risk injuries (e.g., IOFB, rural cases, etc.) may benefit from intravitreal antibiotics.

Oral antibiotics might have good vitreous penetration, but they have limited use in prophylaxis because they may be difficult to administer in patients who cannot take oral medication prior to general anesthesia or if the patient has been nauseated or sedated [38, 75].

Over time several classes of medications have been studied for vitreous penetrance after intravenous administration [75]. Aguilar and colleagues showed in a rabbit study that intravenous ceftazidime achieves much higher vitreous concentrations than MIC levels for *Pseudomonas*, *Streptococcus*, *Klebsiella*, *Serratia*, *E. coli*, and *H. influenza* in inflamed aphakic eyes and similar high concentrations for *Pseudomonas* and other Gram-negative organisms in inflamed phakic eyes. This study suggested that ceftazidime could be used instead of intravenous aminoglycosides for Gram-negative coverage to be used in combination with vancomycin [80]. It is important to remember that ceftazidime has the best coverage for Gram-negative organisms among third-generation cephalosporins but has the least activity against Gram-positive organisms, so it should not be used for adequate coverage [75, 80]. Intravenous prophylaxis can be done with ceftazidime and vancomycin [75]. Andreoli and colleagues reported the lowest endophthalmitis rate (0.9 %) after open-globe injury in 558 patients treated with intravenous vancomycin and ceftazidime (started on admission, stopped after 48 h) [38]. Intravenous prophylaxis with vancomycin and ceftazidime should be strongly considered in all open-globe injuries especially in those with high risk for endophthalmitis.

5.8.2 Intravitreal Prophylaxis

Although intravitreal antibiotics are the most direct method of drug delivery to the eye, toxicity limits their use [81]. Clinically they are often used as an adjunct to systemic therapy. Narang and colleagues compared the combination of intravitreal vancomycin and ceftazidime plus systemic ciprofloxacin with systemic ciprofloxacin only in 70 patients with open-globe injuries. They did not report any statistically significant difference in infection rates, although reported a trend toward improvement with intravitreal injection [60]. Soheilian and colleagues showed in a multicenter, randomized clinical trial that patients who benefit from intravitreal antibiotic prophylaxis were the ones with IOFB [37]. Many authors suggest that intravitreal antibiotics should be used as prophylaxis as an adjunct to systemic therapy only in high-risk cases (e.g., IOFB, rural cases, etc.) [38, 75, 79]. Ceftazidime and vancomycin are the most common choices for prophylactic coverage.

> **Tip**
> Intravitreal antibiotics should be used as prophylaxis as an adjunct to systemic therapy only in high-risk cases (e.g., IOFB, rural cases, etc.).

5.9 Management

Initial treatment of post-traumatic endophthalmitis is empirical and based on symptoms and clinical findings. First line of treatment is intravitreal injection of antibiotics that cover both Gram-positive and Gram-negative organisms. Systemic treatment and other routes should be considered for each patient and causative agent (Tables 5.3 and 5.4). During this initial treatment, samples

Table 5.3 Treatment options and routes of delivery

Route	Medication	Dose
Topical	Vancomycin	50 mg/ml every hour
	Ceftazidime	50 mg/ml every hour
	Gentamicin/tobramycin	14 mg/ml
	Cefazolin	50 mg/ml
	Ciprofloxacin	0.3 % every hour
	Moxifloxacin	0.5 % every hour
	Gatifloxacin	0.3 % every hour
	Topical steroids and cycloplegics should be added	
Subconjunctival	Vancomycin	25 mg
	Ceftazidime	100 mg
	Dexamethasone	12 mg
Oral	Ciprofloxacin	750 mg twice daily
	Levofloxacin	500 mg once daily
	Moxifloxacin	400 mg once daily
	Voriconazole	6 mg/kg/day
	Fluconazole	400–1600 mg/day
Intravenous	Vancomycin	1 g every 12 h
	Ceftazidime	1 g every 8 h
	Amikacin	200–400 μg/ml
	Amphotericin B[a]	0.6–1 mg/kg/day
	Voriconazole	6 mg/kg/day
	Fluconazole	400–1600 mg/day
Intravitreal	Vancomycin	1 mg/0.1 ml
	Ceftazidime	2.25 mg/0.1 ml
	Amikacin	0.4 mg/0.1 ml
	Piperacillin/tazobactam	250 μg/0.1 ml
	Amphotericin B[a]	5 μg/0.1 ml
	Voriconazole	0.05–0.1 mg/0.1 ml
	Dexamethasone	0.4 mg/0.1 ml
Intraocular infusion	Vancomycin	0.2 mg/ml
	Ceftazidime	0.45 mg/ml
	Amikacin	0.08 mg/ml
	Gentamicin/tobramycin	0.08 mg/ml
	Amphotericin B	0.02 mg/ml
	Dexamethasone	0.04–0.08 mg/ml

[a]Amphotericin should be prepared in distilled water or 5 % dextrose not in saline solution

Table 5.4 Preparation of commonly used fortified topical antibiotics

Vancomycin
Dissolve 500 mg vancomycin in 10 ml 0.9 % NaCl (=50 mg/ml)
Ceftazidime
Take 500 mg powder vial and dissolve with 10 ml of artificial teardrops or 0.09 % NaCl
Cefazolin
Take 500 mg powder vial and dissolve with 10 ml of artificial teardrops or 0.09 % NaCl
Preparation of commonly used intravitreal antibiotics
Vancomycin
Dissolve 500 mg vancomycin in 10 ml 0.9 % NaCl (=50 mg/ml) Dilute 2 ml of the solution (=100 mg) with 8 ml of 0.9 % NaCl (=10 mg/ml) Draw in tuberculin syringe for more precise dosage measurement Inject 0.1 ml (1 mg) into midvitreous
Ceftazidime
Take 500 mg powder vial and dissolve with 10 ml 0.09 % NaCl (=50 mg/ml) Dilute 4.5 ml of the solution (=225 mg) with 5.5 ml of 0.09 % NaCl (=22.5 mg/ml) Draw in tuberculin syringe for more precise dosage measurement Inject 0.1 ml (2.25 mg) into midvitreous
Amikacin
Begin with 100 mg vial of amikacin (2 ml) Take 0.8 ml (=40 mg) and dilute with 9.2 ml 0.09 % NaCl (=4 mg/ml) Draw in tuberculin syringe for more precise dosage measurement Inject 0.1 ml (0.4 mg) into midvitreous
Amphotericin B
Dissolve 50 mg amphotericin B in 10 ml aqua or 5 % dextrose (not in 0.09 % NaCl) Take 0.1 ml (=0.5 mg) and dilute with 9.9 ml aqua or 5 % dextrose Draw in tuberculin syringe for more precise dosage measurement Inject 0.1 ml (0.005 mg) into midvitreous
Voriconazole
Dissolve 200 mg voriconazole in 20 ml aqua or 5 % dextrose (NOT in 0.09 % NaCl) Take 1 ml (=10 mg) and dilute with 10 ml aqua or 5 % dextrose (=1 mg/ml) Draw in tuberculin syringe for more precise dosage measurement Inject 0.1 ml (0.005 mg) into midvitreous

are obtained from suitable sites (anterior chamber, vitreous, wound, and conjunctiva) for culture and stains. Once the results are available, treatment should be modified according to the susceptibility of the organisms [8, 9, 60].

5.9.1 Intravitreal Injections

Intravitreal injections give the highest amount of drug delivery into the vitreous compared to other modalities (topical, subconjunctival, intravenous) [82, 83]. The best drug combination is vancomycin (1 mg/0.1 ml) and ceftazidime (2.25 mg/0.1 ml) [60]. Vancomycin covers all Gram-positive organisms and has little resistance. In the Endophthalmitis Vitrectomy Study (EVS), 100% of Gram-positive organisms, including methicillin-resistant *Staphylococcus*, were sensitive to vancomycin [84]. In cases of *Bacillus*, endophthalmitis amikacin (0.4 mg/0.1 ml) can be added to vancomycin.

For the immediate empirical treatment of post-traumatic endophthalmitis, aminoglycosides (e.g., amikacin, gentamicin) should be avoided due to possible retinal toxicity [2, 14, 54, 58, 85]. Some authors recommend the use of amikacin instead of ceftazidime with the following rationale: amikacin has been tested in the prospective EVS trial for its efficacy, it provides concentration-dependent rapid killing of organisms, and it acts synergistically with vancomycin. Ceftazidime, on the other side, can precipitate in the vitreous cavity [54, 86]. But clinicians should keep in mind that in the EVS, all Gram-negative isolates were equally sensitive to amikacin and ceftazidime, and ceftazidime has an excellent safety profile with a possible synergistic effect with vancomycin [54, 58, 87, 88].

> **Tip**
> Vancomycin and ceftazidime should be given in two separate syringes in order not to cause precipitation of antibiotics.

In cases of Gram-negative organisms including *Pseudomonas*, ceftazidime can be used [60]. For *Pseudomonas* endophthalmitis, intravitreal piperacillin/tazobactam (250 µg/0.1 ml) may be used as an alternative to ceftazidime [89].

For fungal infection, intravitreal amphotericin B (5 µ/0.1 ml) has been considered as a golden standard. For lesser side effects, pars plana vitrectomy (PPV) with oral fluconazole has been reported for treating *Candida* endophthalmitis successfully. It has been shown that oral fluconazole has significant penetration into the noninflamed eye [70, 90]. Voriconazole is a second-generation synthetic derivative of fluconazole and has a broad spectrum including *Aspergillus* spp., *Candida* spp., and *Paecilomyces* [70, 91]. Intravitreal use of voriconazole has also been reported to be effective [92, 93].

Intravitreal antibiotics should be prepared in separate injectors to avoid drug precipitation, and each injector should be labeled to avoid confusion. Subconjunctival local anesthetic injection may help the patient during the tap and intravitreal injection. Empirical treatment should be initiated right away. We recommend preparing the patient for tap and injection as soon as possible even if the surgery is planned for the next day.

Following a proper injection and tap procedure, if there is no clinical improvement with close monitoring of the eye (four times a day or hourly), immediate PPV should be considered [9, 28, 94].

5.9.2 Systemic Antibiotics

Although addition of *intravenous antibiotic therapy* to intravitreal antibiotics did not show a clear benefit in the EVS, these results may not be relevant to post-traumatic endophthalmitis for the following reasons [8, 54, 84]:

- EVS included only postoperative endophthalmitis within 6 weeks of surgery, and this causes the microbial spectrum to be different.
- The flaws in EVS study design: although Gram-positive organisms were the most common agents of all growth (94%) in EVS

study, ceftazidime and amikacin were the drugs chosen for intravenous treatment [84]. Approximately 50 % of Gram-positive organisms were resistant to ceftazidime in the EVS [84]. Thus, systemic antibiotics may not have shown additional benefit in treating postoperative endophthalmitis in the EVS because of inappropriate selection of the antibiotics [8, 84].

There are many options for systemic antibiotic treatment. Intravenous vancomycin (1 g every 12 h) and ceftazidime (1 g every 8 h) is one option [2, 60, 95]. Amikacin can be used instead of ceftazidime [96] if a patient is allergic to penicillins or cephalosporins. We prefer intravenous vancomycin 2×1 and ceftazidime 3×1 for the first 2–3 days and continue with oral moxifloxacin 400 mg once a day for a week.

Oral fluoroquinolones (ciprofloxacin and levofloxacin being the third generation and moxifloxacin and gatifloxacin being the fourth generation) can achieve effective vitreous concentrations even in noninflamed eyes. Ciprofloxacin 750 mg bid achieves vitreous concentrations which exceeds MIC90 of *Staphylococcus epidermidis*, *Propionibacterium* spp., *Pseudomonas aeruginosa*, and *Proteus mirabilis* and MIC70 of *Staphylococcus aureus* and *Bacillus cereus* even in noninflamed eyes [55]. Similarly levofloxacin and moxifloxacin can achieve above MIC90 concentrations of most microorganisms known to cause post-traumatic endophthalmitis [56, 57].

Fourth-generation fluoroquinolones (moxifloxacin and gatifloxacin) have better coverage than earlier-generation fluoroquinolones against Gram-positive organisms [57]. Although moxifloxacin and gatifloxacin have similar vitreous penetration in the uninflamed eye, Bristol-Myers Squibb has stopped manufacturing systemic gatifloxacin because of its life-threatening complications such as serious hyperglycemia [97].

Systemic fluoroquinolones were not readily available in the era of EVS; thus there is no prospective randomized clinical study showing the efficacy of oral fluoroquinolones in endophthalmitis. Further studies are still needed.

5.9.3 Topical Antibiotics

Topical antibiotics should be used with intravitreal antibiotics to increase antibiotic concentration in the eye. Fortified antibiotics including vancomycin (50 mg/ml) and ceftazidime (50 mg/ml) administered every hour can be used until the culture results are available [20, 54]. If vancomycin and ceftazidime cannot be used, fortified gentamicin or tobramycin (14 mg/ml) can be used with cefazolin (50 mg/ml) [13]. Instead of fortified antibiotics, clinicians may use topical fluoroquinolones [98]. Topical ciprofloxacin, moxifloxacin, or gatifloxacin may be used one drop every hour while awake [60]. We usually prefer to use topical fortified vancomycin and ceftazidime for the first few days until the clinical picture of endophthalmitis starts to regress and continue with topical moxifloxacin thereafter.

5.9.4 Subconjunctival Antibiotics

Subconjunctival antibiotics may have therapeutic levels especially in the anterior chamber. This should be reserved for patients who cannot administer frequent drops [8].

5.9.5 Steroid Therapy

Steroid therapy is controversial. There is no consensus in the timing, dosing, and the route of administration of steroids in post-traumatic endophthalmitis. Treatment of post-traumatic infection with antibiotics, especially in Gram-negative organisms, leads to further release of endotoxins which can exacerbate the ocular damage [99]. In cases of infections, host inflammatory response can additionally increase the damage. In bacterial endophthalmitis, corticosteroids may be beneficial to control inflammation- and infection-related tissue injuries [99–101]. EVS did not use intravitreal steroids but recommended the use of systemic steroids for acute postoperative endophthalmitis [54]. It is wise to consider the use of intravitreal corticosteroids in bacterial endophthalmitis to eliminate the systemic side effects.

One of the drawbacks of steroid use in post-traumatic endophthalmitis is decreasing host defense against infection. Especially when the organism is not susceptible to the empirical treatment as in fungal endophthalmitis, steroids might contribute to progression of the infection. Some retina specialists defer steroid treatment 12 h after antibiotic administration to allow the effect to take place [8].

There may also be the risk of drug reaction between steroids and antibiotics. Studies have shown that intravitreal dexamethasone may enhance the activity of vancomycin by prolonging the half-life in the vitreous [102, 103]. In a study with 57 postoperative endophthalmitis cases, it has been shown that patients receiving intravitreal dexamethasone have a reduced probability of gaining three lines of visual acuity [104]. However many studies suggest that final visual acuity is independent of steroid use [100, 105].

On the other hand, inflammation control may shorten the duration of endophthalmitis leading to better structural recovery. Overall, the use of intravitreal dexamethasone is a relatively safe management option provided that fungal infection is not present. Dexamethasone clears quickly from the vitreous cavity within 3 days of injection [106]. Dexamethasone doses exceeding 0.8 mg have been found to be toxic to neurosensory retina [106]. We recommend dexamethasone (0.4 mg/0.1 ml) on a routine basis which has been shown to reduce inflammation in a nontoxic dose [22, 54, 95, 100, 106–108].

> **Tip**
>
> Our first line of treatment in endophthalmitis is urgent intravitreal tap and injection of antibiotics (vancomycin and ceftazidime) with addition of intravitreal 0.4 mg/0.1 ml dexamethasone if there is no suspicion of fungal endophthalmitis.

Topical steroids should be started as soon as intravitreal antibiotics are injected. We use prednisolone acetate 1 % drops on an hourly basis while awake until the inflammation starts to subside and then tapered. If fungal infection is suspected, initiation of steroids should be withheld until clear signs of improvement are noted [100]. Topical steroids can be used even for months for the control of residual inflammation following endophthalmitis.

We prefer intravenous vancomycin 2 × 1 and ceftazidime 3 × 1 for the first 2–3 days and continue with oral moxifloxacin 400 mg once a day for a week.

Topical fortified vancomycin and ceftazidime are ordered on an hourly basis during the first 24 h than tapered according to the infection control before switching to moxifloxacin eye drops later.

Topical steroids (prednisolone acetate 1 %) are started after intravitreal injection of antibiotics once every hour while awake and then tapered according to inflammation control. The use of topical steroids might be as long as months to control the inflammation.

5.9.6 Surgery

In post-traumatic endophthalmitis, *pars plana vitrectomy (PPV)* allows treatment of residual intraocular effects of the trauma such as retained lens material, vitreous hemorrhage, retinal breaks, and removal of IOFB, as well as allowing removal of infected vitreous, bacteria, and toxins [9]. The approach to post-traumatic endophthalmitis is different than postoperative endophthalmitis in this respect. If there is IOFB, urgent PPV is imperative. Many authors, like us, suggest early PPV for post-traumatic endophthalmitis even if there is no IOFB [81, 109]. Early intervention will have the advantage of repairing traumatic damage to the eye (e.g., retinal detachment) as well as treatment of endophthalmitis.

In cases of fungal endophthalmitis, it is difficult to clear the infection with antifungals once there is vitreous invasion [9, 81, 95, 109].

After the first injection of antibiotics, the eye should be monitored closely (even hourly) until signs of regression of the infection. If there is no improvement, PPV should be considered regardless of visual acuity [8, 9, 94].

There are different vitrectomy techniques reported. Also extent of the surgery (e.g., removal of posterior hyaloid, use of silicone oil) is controversial [8, 9, 61]. We believe extent of the surgery should be tailored for each patient according to the residual effects of the trauma (e.g., retinal detachment, IOFB) and collateral damage of the infection (e.g., retinitis).

First technical problem is visualization due to corneal edema, anterior chamber inflammation, ruptured lens, and/or vitreous opacities. If necessary corneal epithelium can be scraped, anterior chamber inflammation and fibrin exudates should be excised either with an aspiration probe or a vitrectomy probe (with active irrigation in the anterior chamber), and if the crystalline lens is ruptured, it should be removed (Case 5.3a, b). Infusion port should be entered and used only after one can verify the location of the tip of the infusion in the vitreous cavity. At this stage if the cornea does not allow visualization, a temporary keratoprosthesis can be used followed by a penetrating keratoplasty [9].

Samples from the eye should be obtained early in the case even before activating the infusion line. At this stage using air instead of balanced salt solution might protect the intraocular pressure, without diluting the intraocular contents that are being aspirated.

After core vitrectomy and visualization of the retina, surgeon should decide the extent of the operation. A limited vitrectomy should be planned if the retina is attached, inflamed, and fragile with intraretinal hemorrhages and cotton wool spots. Posterior hyaloid removal can be considered if the retina looks healthy. Posterior hyaloid separation can be attempted, but should not be insisted on it. The inflamed retina is fragile and prone to tears; thus the vitreous should be cleared away as safely as possible. However if there is significant debris under internal limiting membrane (ILM) and retinitis is of low grade (Case 5.2e), ILM peeling may be considered with caution (Case 5.2f).

Tip
When silicone oil is used as a tamponade in PPV, intravitreal antibiotic doses should be reduced by 1/3–1/10.

Silicone oil use as a tamponade after PPV for endophthalmitis is shown to be beneficial when there is rhegmatogenous retinal detachment, when there is a risk of occult retinal tears, and because of its antimicrobial properties [12, 110–113]. We use silicone oil tamponade in all cases of endophthalmitis with significant retinitis even in the absence of retinal breaks because of its antimicrobial properties. The use of air tamponade is another option for those without significant retinitis, which we believe, also, has some anti-inflammatory effect [114].

At the end of the procedure, intravitreal antibiotics should be injected. We use them together with dexamethasone. When silicone oil is used as a tamponade, concentrations of antibiotics and dexamethasone should be reduced by 1/3–1/10 of the normal dose to reduce toxicity. Instead of using intravitreal antibiotics at the end of the case, it is also recommended to use antibiotics in the intraocular infusion (Table 5.3).

Tip
Intraocular injections and intraocular infusions are alternative options; they should not be used together.

If treatment is effective, patients usually have a dramatic decrease in ocular pain within the first postoperative day. Keep in mind that the need for multiple operations is frequent in patients with endophthalmitis. In EVS, 35 % of eyes needed secondary procedures [54].

Conclusion

Endophthalmitis after open-globe injury is the second largest category after postoperative cases accounting for 20–30 % of the endophthalmitis cases, and it remains a devastating complication of ocular trauma. Clinicians should maintain a high suspicion of endophthalmitis after trauma since symptoms and signs of trauma might mask the infection.

In an open-globe injury, immediate wound closure with early treatment with systemic antibiotics may be the best approach to prevent post-traumatic endophthalmitis.

Risk factors for post-traumatic endophthalmitis include IOFB, lens rupture, delayed primary wound repair, large wound size, ocular tissue prolapse, pediatric age group, and rural trauma. If there are multiple risk factors, consider using prophylactic intravitreal antibiotics. Third- and fourth-generation fluoroquinolones cover most of the causative organisms and have good penetration into vitreous cavity when used orally.

Empirical treatment should be started right away. Our first line of treatment is intravitreal vancomycin, ceftazidime, and dexamethasone injections (unless contraindicated). We also add oral fluoroquinolones (ciprofloxacin or moxifloxacin). If organic matter is the cause of the trauma and the presenting symptoms are indolent, fungal endophthalmitis should be suspected and treated with intravitreal amphotericin B and/or intravenous voriconazole.

There are still many controversies with respect to route of antibiotic prophylaxis, intravitreal use of steroids, surgical timing, extent of vitrectomy, and the role of silicone oil. It is very difficult to adopt a treatment schedule for every case because every post-traumatic endophthalmitis is unique depending on the extent of injury and virulence of the infective organism. Every case should be considered separately, and more prospective controlled studies are needed to conclude.

References

1. McGwin Jr G, Xie A, Owsley C. Rate of eye injury in the United States. Arch Ophthalmol. 2005;123:970–6.
2. Danis RP. Endophthalmitis. Ophthalmol Clin North Am. 2002;15(2):243–8.
3. Parrish CM, O'Day DM. Traumatic endophthalmitis. Int Ophthalmol Clin. 1987;27(2):112–9.
4. Verbracken H, Rysselaere M. Post-traumatic endophthalmitis. Eur J Ophthalmol. 1994;4(1):1–5.
5. Kuhn F, Morris R, Witherspoon CD, Heimann K, Jeffers JB, Treister G. A standardized classification of ocular trauma. Ophthalmology. 1996;103:240–3.
6. Kuhn F, Morris R, Witherspoon CD. Birmingham Eye Trauma Terminology (BETT): terminology and classification of mechanical eye injuries. Ophthalmol Clin North Am. 2002;15:139–43.
7. Schrader WF. Open globe injuries: epidemiological study of two eye clinics in Germany, 1981–1999. Croat Med J. 2004;45:268–74.
8. Bhagat N, Nagori S, Zarbin M. Post-traumatic infectious endophthalmitis. Surv Ophthalmol. 2011;56:214–51.
9. Meredith TA, Ulrich JN. Infectious endophthalmitis. In: Ryan SJ, Wilkinson CP, Wiedeman P, editors. Retina. 5th ed. New York, Elsevier-Saunders; 2013. p. 2019–39.
10. Thompson JT, Parver LM, Enger CL, Mieler WF, Liggett PE. Infectious endophthalmitis after penetrating injuries with retained intraocular foreign bodes. National Eye Trauma System. Ophthalmology. 1993;100:1468–74.
11. Jonas JB, Knorr HLJ, Budde WM. Prognostic factors in ocular injuries caused by intraocular or retrobulbar foreign bodies. Ophthalmology. 2000;107:823–8.
12. Azad R, Ravi K, Talwar D, Rajpal, Kumar N. Pars plana vitrectomy with or without silicone oil endotamponade in post-traumatic endophthalmitis. Graefes Arch Clin Exp Ophthalmol. 2003;241:478–83.
13. Brinton GS, Topping TM, Hyndiuk RA, Aaberg TM, Reeser FH, Abrams GW. Posttraumatic endophthalmitis. Arch Ophthalmol. 1984;102:547–50.
14. Essex RW, Yi Q, Charles PG, Allen PG. Post-traumatic endophthalmitis. Ophthalmology. 2004;111:2015–22.
15. Boldt HC, Pulido JS, Blodi CF, Folk JC, Weingeist TA. Rural endophthalmitis. Ophthalmology. 1989;96:1722–6.
16. Ariyasu RG, Kumar S, LaBree LD, Wagner DG, Smith RE. Microorganisms cultured from the anterior chamber of ruptured globes at the time of repair. Am J Ophthalmol. 1995;119:181–8.
17. Behrens-Baumann W, Praetorius G. Intraocular foreign bodies, 297 consecutive cases. Ophthalmologica. 1989;198:84–8.
18. Mieler WF, Ellis MK, Williams DF. Retained intraocular foreign bodies and endophthalmitis. Ophthalmology. 1990;97:1532–8.
19. Rubsamen PE, Cousins SW, Martinez JA. Impact of cultures on management decisions following surgical repair of penetrating ocular trauma. Ophthalmic Surg Lasers. 1997;28:43–9.
20. Ahmed Y, Schimel AM, Pathengay A, Colyer MH, Flynn Jr HW. Endophthalmitis following open-globe injuries. Eye. 2012;26:212–7.
21. Alfaro DV, Roth DB, Liggett PE. Posttraumatic endophthalmitis. Causative organisms, treatment, and prevention. Retina. 1994;14:206–11.

22. Reynolds DS, Flynn Jr HW. Endophthalmitis after penetrating ocular trauma. Curr Opin Ophthalmol. 1997;8:32–8.
23. Peyman GA, Carroll CP, Raichand M. Prevention and management of traumatic endophthalmitis. Ophthalmology. 1980;87:320–4.
24. Williams DF, Mieler WF, Abrams GW, et al. Results and prognostic factors in penetrating ocular injuries with retained intraocular foreign bodies. Ophthalmology. 1988;95:911–6.
25. Sugar AM. Agents of mucormycosis and related species. In: Mandell GL, Bennett JE, Dolin R, editors. Principles and practice of infectious diseases. 6th ed. Philedelphia, PA: Elsevier, Churchill, Livingstone;2005:2973–84.
26. Vedantham V, Nirmalan PK, Ramasamy K, et al. Clinicomicrobiological profile and visual outcomes of posttraumatic endophthalmitis at a tertiary eye care center in South India. Indian J Ophthalmol. 2006;54(1):5–10.
27. Ferrer C, Montero J, Alio JL, et al. Rapid molecular diagnosis of posttraumatic keratitis and endophthalmitis caused by Alternaria infectoria. J Clin Microbiol. 2003;41:3358–60.
28. Lee SY, Ryan SJ. Pathophysiology of ocular trauma. In: Ryan SJ, Wilkinson CP, Wiedeman P, editors. Retina. 5th ed. New York, Elsevier-Saunders; 2013. p. 1647–55.
29. Cebulla CM, Flynn Jr HW. Endophthalmitis after open globe injuries. Am J Ophthalmol. 2009;147:567–8.
30. Ferrari TM, Cardascia N, Di Gesu I, et al. Early versus late removal of retained intraocular foreign bodies. Retina. 2001;21:92–3.
31. Mester V, Kuhn F. Intraocular foreign bodies. Ophthalmol Clin North Am. 2002;15:235–42.
32. Tawara A. Transformation and cytotoxicity of iron in siderosis bulbi. Invest Ophthalmol Vis Sci. 1986;27:226–36.
33. Knave B. Long-term changes in retinal function induced by short, high intensity flashes. Experientia. 1969;25:379–80.
34. Colyer MH, Chun DW, Bower KS, et al. Perforating globe injuries during operation Iraqi Freedom. Ophthalmology. 2008;115:2087–93.
35. Zhang Y, Zhang M, Jiang C, et al. Endophthalmitis following open globe injury. Br J Ophthalmol. 2010;94:111–4.
36. Meredith TA. Posttraumatic endophthalmitis. Arch Ophthalmol. 1999;117:520–1.
37. Soheilian M, Rafati N, Mohebbi MR, et al. Prophylaxis of acute posttraumatic bacterial endophthalmitis: a multicenter, randomized clinical trial of intraocular antibiotic injection, report 2. Arch Ophthalmol. 2007;125:460–5.
38. Andreoli CM, Andreoli MT, Kloek CE, et al. Low rate of endophthalmitis in a large series of open globe injuries. Am J Ophthalmol. 2009;147:601–8.e2.
39. Gupta A, Srinivasan R, Gulnar D, et al. Risk factors for post-traumatic endophthalmitis in patients with positive intraocular cultures. Eur J Ophthalmol. 2007;17:642–7.
40. Duch-Samper AM, Menezo JL, Hurtado-Sarrio M. Endophthalmitis following penetrating eye injuries. Acta Ophthalmol Scand. 1997;75:104–6.
41. Recchia FM, Sternberg P. Surgery for ocular trauma: principles and techniques of treatment. In: Ryan SJ, Wilkinson CP, Wiedeman P, editors. Retina. 5th ed. New York, Elsevier-Saunders; 2013. p. 1852–75.
42. Dehghani AR, Rezai L, Salam H, Mohammadi Z, Mahboubi M. Post traumatic endophthalmitis: incidence and risk factors. Glob J Health Sci. 2014;6:68–72.
43. Narang S, Gupta V, Simalandhi P, Gupta A, Raj S, Dogra MR. Paediatric open globe injuries. Visual outcome and risk factors for endophthalmitis. Indian J Ophthalmol. 2004;52:29–34.
44. Li X, Zarbin MA, Bhagat N. Pediatric open globe injury: a review of the literature. J Emerg Trauma Shock. 2015;8:201–23.
45. Scharf J, Zonis S. Perforating injuries of the eye in childhood. J Pediatr Ophthalmol. 1976;13:326–8.
46. Alfaro DV, Roth DB, Laughlin RM, et al. Paediatric posttraumatic endophthalmitis. Br J Ophthalmol. 1995;79:888–91.
47. Jalali S, Das T, Majji AB. Hypodermic needles: a new source of penetrating ocular trauma in Indian children. Retina. 1999;19:213–7.
48. Junejo SA, Ahmet M, Alam M. Endophthalmitis in paediatric penetrating ocular injuries in Hyderabad. J Pak Med Assoc. 2010;60:532–5.
49. Hosseini H, Masoumpour M, Keshavarz-Fazl F, Razeghinejad MR, Salouti R, Nowroozzadeh MH. Clinical and epidemiologic characteristics of severe childhood ocular injuries in Southern Iran. Middle East Afr J Ophthalmol. 2011;18:136–40.
50. Castellarin AA, Pieramici DJ. Open globe management. Compr Ophthalmol Update. 2007;8:11–24.
51. Sul S, Gurelik G, Korkmaz S, Ozdek S, Hasanreisoglu B. Pediatric open-globe injuries: clinical characteristics and factors associated with poor visual and anatomical success. Graefes Arch Clin Exp Ophthalmol. 2015;254(7):1405–10.
52. Chhabra S, Kunimoto DY, Kazi L, et al. Endophthalmitis after open globe injury: microbiologic spectrum and susceptibilities of isolates. Am J Ophthalmol. 2006;142:852–4.
53. Sabaci G, Bayer A, Mutlu FM, et al. Endophthalmitis after deadly-weapon-related open-globe injuries: risk factors, value of prophylactic antibiotics, and visual outcomes. Am J Ophthalmol. 2002;133:62–9.
54. Results of the Endophthalmitis Vitrectomy Study. A randomized trial of immediate vitrectomy and of intravenous antibiotics for the treatment of postoperative bacterial endophthalmitis. Endophthalmitis Vitrectomy Study Group. Arch Ophthalmol 1995;113:1479–96.
55. Lesk MR, Ammann H, Marcil G, et al. The penetration of oral ciprofloxacin into the aqueous humor, vitreous, and subretinal fluid of humans. Am J Ophthalmol. 1993;115:623–8.
56. Garcia-Saenz MC, Arias-Puente A, Fresnadillo-Martinez MJ, et al. Human aqueous humor levels of

oral ciprofloxacin, levofloxacin, and moxifloxacin. J Cataract Refract Surg. 2001;27:1969–74.
57. Hariprasad SM, Shah GK, Mieler WF, et al. Vitreous and aqueous penetration of orally administered moxifloxacin in humans. Arch Ophthalmol. 2006;124:178–82.
58. Galloway G, Ramsay A, Jordan K, et al. Macular infarction after intravitreal amikacin: mounting evidence against amikacin. Br J Ophthalmol. 2002;86:359–60.
59. Lieb DF, Scott IU, Flynn Jr HW, et al. Open globe injuries with positive intraocular cultures: factors influencing final visual acuity outcomes. Ophthalmology. 2003;110:1560–6.
60. Narang S, Gupta V, Gupta A, et al. Role of prophylactic intravitreal antibiotics in open globe injuries. Indian J Ophthalmol. 2003;51:39–44.
61. Abu el-Asrar AM, Tabbara KF. Clostridium perfringens endophthalmitis. Doc Ophthalmol. 1994;87:177–82.
62. La Cour M, Norgaard A, Prause JU, et al. Gas gangrene panophthalmitis. A case from Greenland. Acta Ophthalmol (Copenh). 1994;72:524–8.
63. Wilk CM, Ruprecht KW, Lang GK. Fulminant gas gangrene panophthalmia following perforating scleral injury. Klin Monatsbl Augenheilkd. 1989;195:243–7.
64. Kelly LD, Steahly LP. Successful prophylaxis of Clostridium perfringens endophthalmitis. Arch Ophthalmol. 1991;109:1199.
65. Kunimoto DY, Das T, Sharma S, et al. Microbiologic spectrum and susceptibility of isolates: part II. Posttraumatic endophthalmitis. Endophthalmitis Research Group. Am J Ophthalmol. 1999;128:242–4.
66. Tran TP, Le TM, Bui HT, et al. Post-traumatic endophthalmitis after penetrating injury in Vietnam: risk factors, microbiological aspect and visual outcome. Klin Monatsbl Augenheilkd. 2003;220:481–5.
67. Iyer MN, Kranias G, Daun ME. Post-traumatic endophthalmitis involving Clostridium tetani and Bacillus spp. Am J Ophthalmol. 2001;132(1):116–7.
68. Rowsey JJ, Newsom DL, Sexton DJ, et al. Endophthalmitis: current approaches. Ophthalmology. 1982;89:1055–66.
69. Wykoff CC, Flynn Jr HW, Miller D, Scott IU, Alfonso EC. Exogenous fungal endophthalmitis: microbiology and clinical outcomes. Ophthalmology. 2008;115(9):1501–7.
70. Kalkanci A, Ozdek S, Ozmen MC. Ocular fungal infections. 1st ed. Saarbrücken: Germany, Lambert Academic Publishing; 2015.
71. Pflugfelder SC, Flynn Jr HW, Zwickey TA, et al. Exogenous fungal endophthalmitis. Ophthalmology. 1988;95:19–30.
72. Kuhn F, Maisiak R, Mann L, et al. The ocular trauma score (OTS). Ophthalmol Clin North Am. 2002;15:163–5, vi.
73. Nelsen PT, Marcus DA, Bovino JA. Retinal detachment following endophthalmitis. Ophthalmology. 1985;92:1112–7.
74. Affeldt JC, Flynn Jr HW, Forster RK, et al. Microbial endophthalmitis resulting from ocular trauma. Ophthalmology. 1987;94:407–13.
75. Lorch A, Sobrin L. Prophylactic antibiotics in posttraumatic infectious endophthalmitis. Int Ophthalmol Clinics. 2013;53:167–76.
76. Alfaro DV, Pince K, Park J, et al. Systemic antibiotics prophylaxis in penetrating ocular injuries. An experimental study. Retina. 1992;12:S3–6.
77. Fiscella RG, Nguyen TK, Cwik MJ, et al. Aqueous and vitreous penetration of levofloxacin after oral administration. Ophthalmology. 1999;106:2286–90.
78. Herbert EN, Pearce IA, McGalliard J, et al. Vitreous penetration of levofloxacin in the uninflamed phakic human eye. Br J Ophthalmol. 2002;86:387–9.
79. Woodcock MG, Scott RA, Huntbach J, et al. Mass and shape as factors in intraocular foreign body injuries. Ophthalmology. 2006;113:2262–9.
80. Aguilar HE, Meredith TA, Shaarawy A, et al. Vitreous cavity penetration of ceftazidime after intravenous administration. Retina. 1995;15:154–9.
81. Mittra RA, Mieler WF. Controversies in the management of open-globe injuries involving the posterior segment. Surv Ophthalmol. 1999;44:215–25.
82. Baum J, Peyman GA, Barza M. Intravitreal administration of antibiotic in the treatment of bacterial endophthalmitis. III. Consensus. Surv Ophthalmol. 1982;26:204–6.
83. Peyman GA, Vastine DW, Meisels HI. The experimental and clinical use of intravitreal antibiotics to treat bacterial and fungal endophthalmitis. Doc Ophthalmol. 1975;39:183–201.
84. Han DP, Wisniewski SR, Wilson LA, et al. Spectrum and susceptibilities of microbiologic isolates in the Endophthalmitis Vitrectomy Study. AmJ Ophthalmol. 1996;122:1–17.
85. Galloway GD, Ramsay A, Jordan K, et al. Macular infarction after intravitreal amikacin: authors' reply. Br J Ophthalmol. 2004;88:1228.
86. Doft BH, Barza M. Macular infarction after intravitreal amikacin. Br J Ophthalmol. 2004;88:850.
87. Jackson TL, Williamson TH. Amikacin retinal toxicity. Br J Ophthalmol. 1999;83:1199–200.
88. Simon C, Littschwager G. In vitro activity of ceftazidime in combination with other antibiotics. Infection. 1985;13:184–9.
89. Mathau A, Sangwan VS, Pathengay A. Acute postoperative multidrug resistant Pseudomonas aeruginosa endophthalmitis treated with intravitreal piperacillin/tazobactam. Asian J Ophthalmol. 2007;9:185–7.
90. O'Day DM, Foulds G, Williams TE, et al. Ocular uptake of fluconazole following oral administration. Arch Ophthalmol. 1990;108:1006–8.
91. Hariprasad SM, Mieler WF, Holz ER, et al. Determination of vitreous, aqueous, and plasma concentration of orally administered voriconazole in humans. Arch Ophthalmol. 2004;122:42–7.
92. Breit SM, Hariprasad SM, Mieler WF, et al. Management of endogenous fungal endophthalmitis

with voriconazole and caspofungin. Am J Ophthalmol. 2005;139:135–40.
93. Gao H, Pennesi M, Shah K, et al. Safety of intravitreal voriconazole: electroretinographic and histopathologic studies. Trans Am Ophthalmol Soc. 2003;101:183–9.
94. Doft BH, Kelsey SF, Wisniewski SR. Additional procedures after the initial vitrectomy or tap-biopsy in the Endophthalmitis Vitrectomy Study. Ophthalmology. 1998;105:707–16.
95. Kresloff MS, Castellarin AA, Zarbin MA. Endophthalmitis. Surv Ophthalmol. 1998;43: 193–224.
96. Benz MS, Scott IU, Flynn Jr HW, et al. Endophthalmitis isolates and antibiotic sensitivities: a 6-year review of culture-proven cases. Am J Ophthalmol. 2004;137:38–42.
97. Park-Wyllie LY, Juurlink DN, Kopp A, et al. Outpatient gatifloxacin therapy and dysglycemia in older adults. N Engl J Med. 2006;354:1352–61.
98. Aliprandis E, Ciralsky J, Lai H, et al. Comparative efficacy of topical moxifloxacin versus ciprofloxacin and vancomycin in the treatment of P. aeruginosa and ciprofloxacin resistant MRSA keratitis in rabbits. Cornea. 2005;24:201–5.
99. Schulman JA, Peyman GA. Intravitreal corticosteroids as an adjunct in the treatment of bacterial and fungal endophthalmitis. A review. Retina. 1992;12:336–40.
100. Das T, Dogra MR, Gopal L, et al. Postsurgical endophthalmitis: diagnosis and management. Indian J Ophthalmol. 1995;43:103–16.
101. Park SS, Samiy N, Ruoff K, et al. Effect of intravitreal dexamethasone in treatment of pneumococcal endophthalmitis in rabbits. Arch Ophthalmol. 1995;113:1324–9.
102. Gan IM, Ugahary LC, van Dissel JT, et al. Effect of intravitreal dexamethasone on vitreous vancomycin concentrations in patients with suspected postoperative bacterial endophthalmitis. Graefes Arch Clin Exp Ophthalmol. 2005;243:1186–9.
103. Park SS, Vallar RV, Hong CH, et al. Intravitreal dexamethasone effect on intravitreal vancomycin elimination in endophthalmitis. Arch Ophthalmol. 1999;117:1058–62.
104. Shah GK, Stein JD, Sharma S, et al. Visual outcomes following the use of intravitreal steroids in the treatment of postoperative endophthalmitis. Ophthalmology. 2000;107:486–9.
105. Das T, Jalali S, Gothwal VK, et al. Intravitreal dexamethasone in exogenous bacterial endophthalmitis: results of a prospective randomised study. Br J Ophthalmol. 1999;83:1050–5.
106. Kwak HW, D'Amico DJ. Evaluation of the retinal toxicity and pharmacokinetics of dexamethasone after intravitreal injection. Arch Ophthalmol. 1992;110:259–66.
107. Chalam KV, Malkani S, Shah VA. Intravitreal dexamethasone effectively reduces postoperative inflammation after vitreoretinal surgery. Ophthalmic Surg Lasers Imaging. 2003;34:188–92.
108. Duch-Samper AM, Chaques-Alepuz V, Menezo JL, et al. Endophthalmitis following open-globe injuries. Curr Opin Ophthalmol. 1998;9:59–65.
109. Mieler WF, Mittra RA. The role and timing of pars plana vitrectomy in penetrating ocular trauma. Arch Ophthalmol. 1997;115:1191–2.
110. Bali E, Huyghe P, Caspers L, et al. Vitrectomy and silicone oil in the treatment of acute endophthalmitis. Preliminary results. Bull Soc Belge Ophtalmol. 2003;288:9–14.
111. Siqueira RC, Gil AD, Canamary F, et al. Pars plana vitrectomy and silicone oil tamponade for acute endophthalmitis treatment. Arq Bras Oftalmol. 2009;72:28–32.
112. Ozdamar A, Aras C, Ozturk R, et al. In vitro antimicrobial activity of silicone oil against endophthalmitis-causing agents. Retina. 1999;19:122–6.
113. Yan H, Lu Y, Yu J, et al. Silicone oil in the surgical treatment of traumatic endophthalmitis. Eur J Ophthalmol. 2008;18:680–4.
114. Demirci G, Karabas L, Maral H, Ozdek S, Gulkilik G. Effect of air bubble on inflammation after cataract surgery in rabbit eyes. Indian J Ophthalmol. 2013;61:343–8.

Mechanical Ocular Trauma in Children

6

Gokhan Gurelik and Sabahattin Sul

6.1 Introduction

Ocular trauma is the major cause of unilateral blindness in children [1, 2]. Seven to thirteen percent of the patients who suffer from ocular trauma have a significant lower vision and blindness [3, 4]. Thirty-five percent of approximately 2.5 million ocular injuries were encountered in children younger than 17 years old [4]. In Nepal, incidence of ocular trauma (cases that did not require hospitalization were included) was estimated as 300 per 100,000 per year [5]. The incidence of hospitalization due to ocular trauma varies from 8.85 to 22.5 per 100,000 per year [6, 7].

Pediatric ocular trauma does not receive accurate attention even if it is the most common cause of acquired blindness (Fig. 6.1). Approaching and the management of pediatric cases resemble to those in adult cases; nevertheless, pediatric ocular trauma has unique features different from adult ocular trauma. Documenting a reliable history and mechanism of trauma and performing ocular examination are difficult in an injured child. Furthermore, ocular trauma usually affects an immature visual system that is expected to develop up to 9 years old; in other words, amblyopia becomes a major concern following the initial treatment of trauma [8, 9]. Therefore, approaching to ocular trauma in children is different from the adults in some ways and requires special attention.

In this chapter, we described the epidemiological and clinical characteristics, hot topics in the current understanding, current consensuses, controversial areas, and treatment of mechanical ocular trauma in children.

6.2 Epidemiological and Clinical Characteristics of Mechanical Ocular Trauma in Children

Ocular trauma may affect children at any age but peak incidence is about 5–9 years [10]. Boys are affected about two or four times more than girls [11, 12]. Ocular trauma generally occurs at home [10, 11, 13]. In our study representing 182 pediatric open globe injuries in Turkish population, 45.1 % of injuries occur at home [12]. Particularly, infants and younger children are at great risk at home without adult supervision. Furthermore, immature motor-mental skills, carelessness, and uncontrolled emotions increase the rate of home injuries in younger children [6]. The incidence rate of outdoor places such as streets and roads and school tends to increase in older children [13].

G. Gurelik, MD (✉)
Department of Ophthalmology, School of Medicine, Gazi University, Ankara, Turkey
e-mail: gurelik@roketmail.com

S. Sul, MD
Department of Ophthalmology, School of Medicine, S Kocman University, Mugla, Turkey

H. Yan (ed.), *Mechanical Ocular Trauma*, DOI 10.1007/978-981-10-2150-3_6

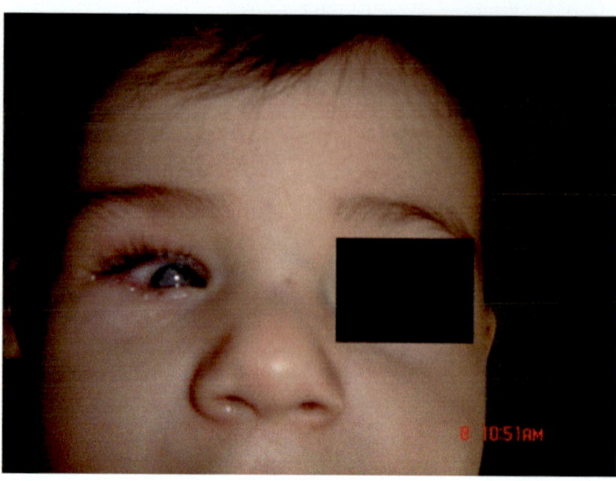

Fig. 6.1 Ocular injury in a baby: a suspicious history of trauma involving both anterior and posterior segment that have resulted in some degree of phthisis bulbi

6.2.1 Environment and Injury Sources

Ocular injuries are commonly accidental compared to those caused by violent assaults and work-related injuries in adults. In general, injuries occur while the child is playing or in sports activity [1, 14]. Accidental falls and blows, hand or finger nail, or toys are the common injury sources in younger children [15–17]. Injuries due to sports account for 27 % of all pediatric ocular trauma that requires hospital admission, and the rate of these injuries increase in older children [1]. In a study from Taiwan, sharp objects (39.8 %) were the common causes of ocular injury [18]. Incidence of projectile-related eye injuries is increasing in the last years due to lack of eyewear protection or adult supervision. Projectiles such as thrown objects (25.2 %) and toy gun bullets (23.1 %) were the major etiologic agents of severe ocular injuries in Greece [19]. Visual outcomes of projectile-related injuries are poor particularly in paintball or air gun injuries and firework-related injuries [20–22]. Listman reported that 43 % of children had a final visual acuity less than 20/200 after paintball injury [20]. Sternberg et al. reported that 59 % of the cases injured with BB pellets required enucleation or evisceration [21]. About 20 years ago, firework (all kinds of explosive agents)-related ocular injuries were creating a burst incidence during especially at short-term festival-like holidays in Turkish children. Nowadays, this kind of injuries occurs very rare after rigid prohibition of explosives by law. Injuries caused by animal attacks (rooster attack, dog bite) or fish hook are prevalent in rural areas [23–25]. Furthermore, hypodermic needle injuries are surprisingly frequent in children [26].

6.2.2 Mechanism of Injury

Almost all ocular injuries occur by direct mechanical effect. Other rare causes of ocular injuries are indirect effects of head or body trauma. Terson's syndrome and shaken baby syndrome are well-known indirect causes of ocular injuries (Fig. 6.2a, b).

Mechanical ocular injuries may be open or closed globe injuries. Closed globe injuries constitute the largest part of the mechanical injuries [13]. Closed globe injuries may be caused by blunt object (contusion), partial laceration with sharp object (lamellar laceration) (Fig. 6.3), and superficial foreign body. Most of the closed globe injuries do not require hospitalization or surgical intervention and have a favorable outcome compared to open globe injuries.

Open globe injuries are encountered 27–48 % of all pediatric ocular injuries [27–31]. Incidence rates increase in hospital-based studies or cases requiring surgical intervention [12, 32]. Open globe injuries constitute of rupture, penetrating injury, perforating injury, and intraocular foreign body according to the Birmingham Eye Trauma Terminology [33]. Penetrating injuries are the most common mechanism in open globe injuries [8, 34]. Anterior and posterior segments are insulted at the same time at almost half of these injuries [35] (Fig. 6.4). Globe ruptures are encountered 9–17 % of the cases in open globe injuries, but the visual outcomes seem to be poor compared to penetrating injuries [8, 28, 36, 37].

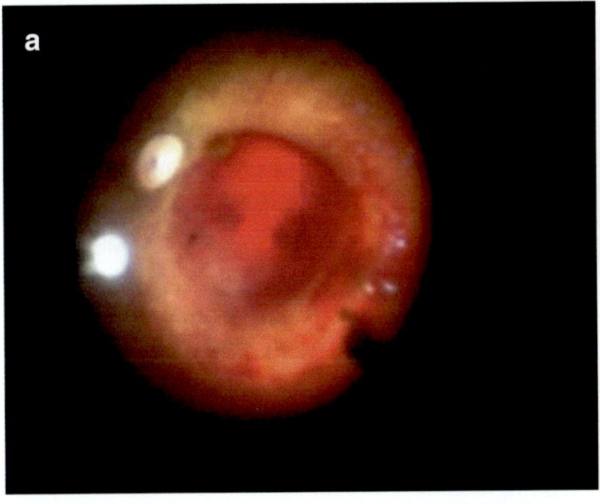

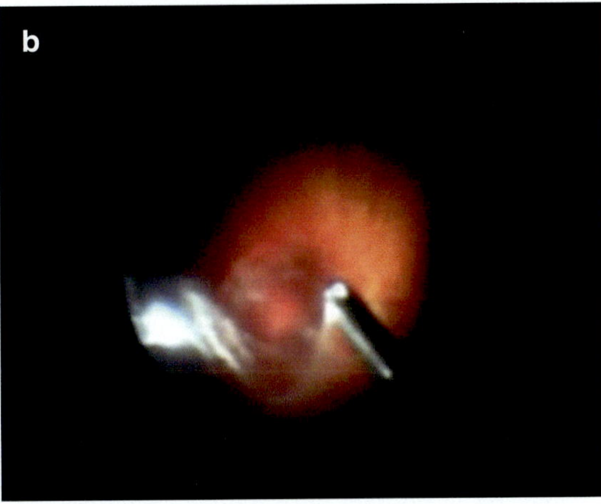

Fig. 6.2 (**a**, **b**) Bilateral indirect ocular injury in a toddler: an 8-month-old baby had visual loss, nystagmus, vitreous hemorrhage, premacular sub-ILM hemorrhage, and optic atrophy in both eyes after a traffic accident 2 months ago. The baby was hospitalized for intracranial, subarachnoid hemorrhage before referral to the eye department. A successful bilateral vitrectomy and ILM peeling were performed to clean premacular hemorrhage. Although rate of nystagmus was diminished, visual acuity gain was limited after the surgery because of bilateral optic atrophy that may be related to intracranial hemorrhage

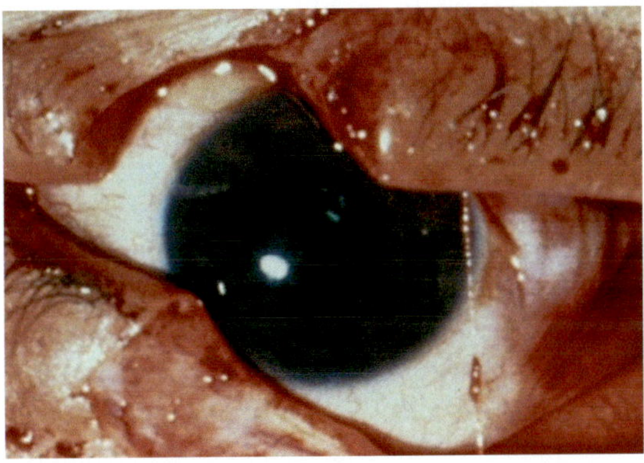

Fig. 6.3 Closed globe injury: sharp object induced lid laceration and lamellar scleral incision

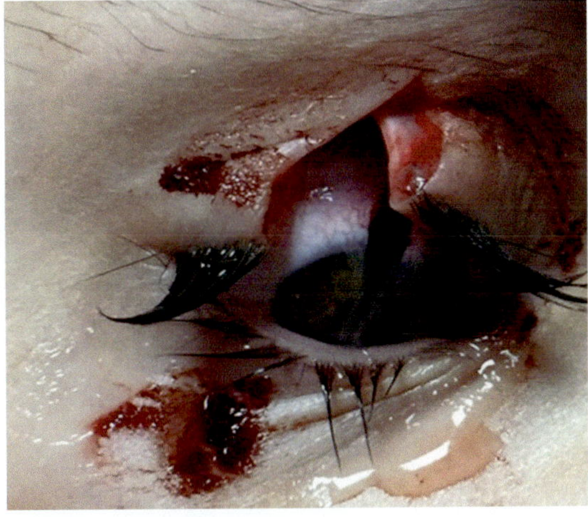

Fig. 6.4 Sharp object induced periocular lid laceration and open globe injury in an 8-year-old boy; corneoscleral incision and involvement of anterior segment structures; iris, lens, and ciliary body

6.3 Evaluation

6.3.1 History

- Taking a reliable history from a child is difficult because:
  - Most of the injuries are not witnessed.
  - Child may not realize visual loss.
  - Child may be distressed and uncooperative.
  - Child may feel itself responsible for the accident and may be afraid of parents' retribution or punishment.

History of the ocular injury should be thorough and preferably taken from the child and includes:

- Time of the injury (important for open globe injuries).

  - Place of the injury.
  - Mechanism of injury (blunt or sharp object, possibility of retained intraocular foreign body).
  - Any change of vision.
  - Any intervention at the time of or after the initial injury.
  - Past medical and ocular history.
  - Injury with an animal bite is more common in children and requires tetanus or rabies prophylaxis.
- It is very important not to remove superficially observed foreign bodies, those that may be in contact with ocular structures or have ocular penetrations out of operation room. Otherwise, ocular tissues may be damaged while removing foreign body or leaking wound may induce further tissue prolapses.
- Eye protection with a sterile eye pad until the surgery is not necessary if there exist large foreign bodies those are superficially exposed as seen in Fig. 6.5.

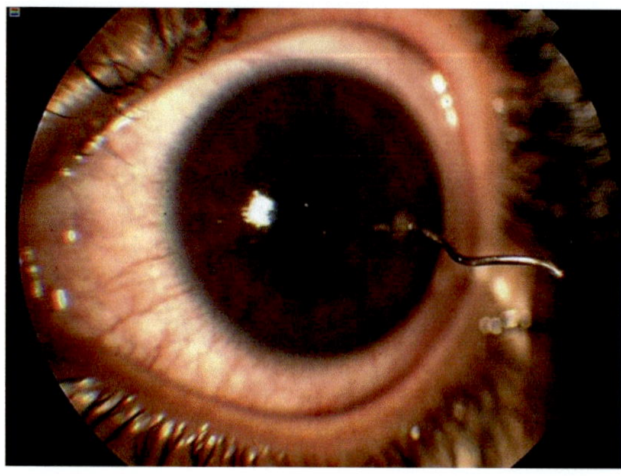

Fig. 6.5 Open globe injury with visible foreign body: a 12-year-old boy was exposed to ocular injury while working at a car repair facility. A piece of wire was responsible from the injury, and one end of the wire was in the anterior chamber. Luckily the body was transferred to our clinic by the help of two other elderly workers keeping the lids open without touching the foreign body. He was taken to the operating room immediately, and corneal repair and foreign body removal were performed. No other tissue damage was noted during the operation, and the eye had 20/20 vision during the follow-up

6.3.2 Examination

- Examination should be quick to determine the extent and management planning of the injury.
- In noncompliant children, examination may be performed under general anesthesia.
- Parents may be asked to assist the examination because the child may be distressed or uncooperative and resist the examination [38].
- Examination starts with a quick inspection of the lids, the adnexa, and the globe for determining wounds, tissue prolapse, chemosis, hemorrhage, and superficial or protruding foreign bodies.
- *Initial visual acuity*:
  - It is important for the prognosis of injury, but unfortunately in small-aged, noncompliant children, that is frequently not possible. Also in open globe injuries involving the cornea, correct visual acuity examination is rarely possible.
  - It should be assessed in each eye separately in age-appropriate manner (Snellen or ETDRS chart for school-going children, E charts for preschool children, and fixation and follow for infants).
  - In the presence of no light perception, electrophysiological tests (ERG/VEP) may be performed in order to evaluate visual integrity. It is also important to remember that negative ERG/VEP responses are not an indication for enucleation or evisceration.
- *Pupil*:
  - Direct and indirect light reflexes
  - The presence or absence of relative afferent pupillary defect (important for prognosis, the presence of associated traumatic optic neuropathy or severe retinal injury)
  - Shape of pupil (any retraction of the pupil may indicate the presence of open globe injury)
- *Intraocular pressure (IOP)*:
  - Low IOP may indicate an underlying open globe injury.

Note: IOP may be normal or elevated especially if the leaking wound is obstructed by the prolapsing intraocular tissues in a case of OGI.

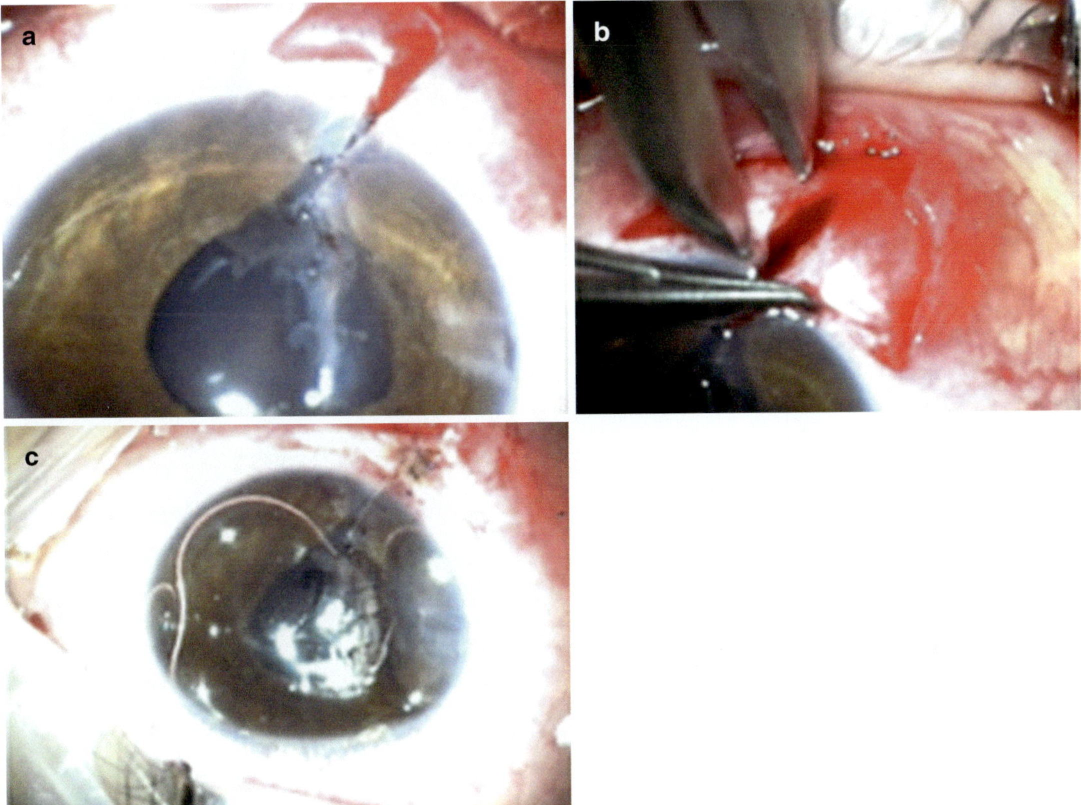

Fig. 6.6 (**a**) Open globe injury with a sharp point kitchen knife in a 4-year-old boy. A corneoscleral wound with deeper penetration involving the iris and lens damage is clearly seen. (**b**) Measuring posterior scleral extension of the wound is crucial during the operation. (**c**) Corneoscleral saturation and reforming anterior chamber with air. Postoperative evaluation showed dense vitreous hemorrhage, retina and choroidal cut, and detachment posteriorly

- *Extent and the length of the wound*:
  - Injuries extending more posterior and wounds greater than 10 mm are associated with poor visual prognosis and high risk of RD development [39, 40] (Fig. 6.6a–c).
- Scleral wound that is not extending more than 5 mm from the limbus does not always indicate survival of the retina. Sharp objects with anteroposterior directional forces frequently touch posterior retina-choroid once it penetrates anterior eyewall in children. Smaller axial length in children may be an additional factor for this situation.
- *Evaluation of vitreous, retina, and choroid.*
- If posterior segment examination is difficult owing to media opacities, diagnostic tests such as ocular USG may be deferred after primary open globe repair (Fig. 6.7a, b).
- At the time of OGI, orbital CT may be sometimes helpful in order to diagnose choroidal detachment before primary open globe repair (Fig. 6.7c).

6.4 Anterior Segment Injuries and Management

- *Subconjunctival hemorrhage*:
  - In adult population, spontaneous subconjunctival hemorrhage may occur without ocular trauma, and conversely in childhood, spontaneous subconjunctival hemorrhage is extremely rare so that

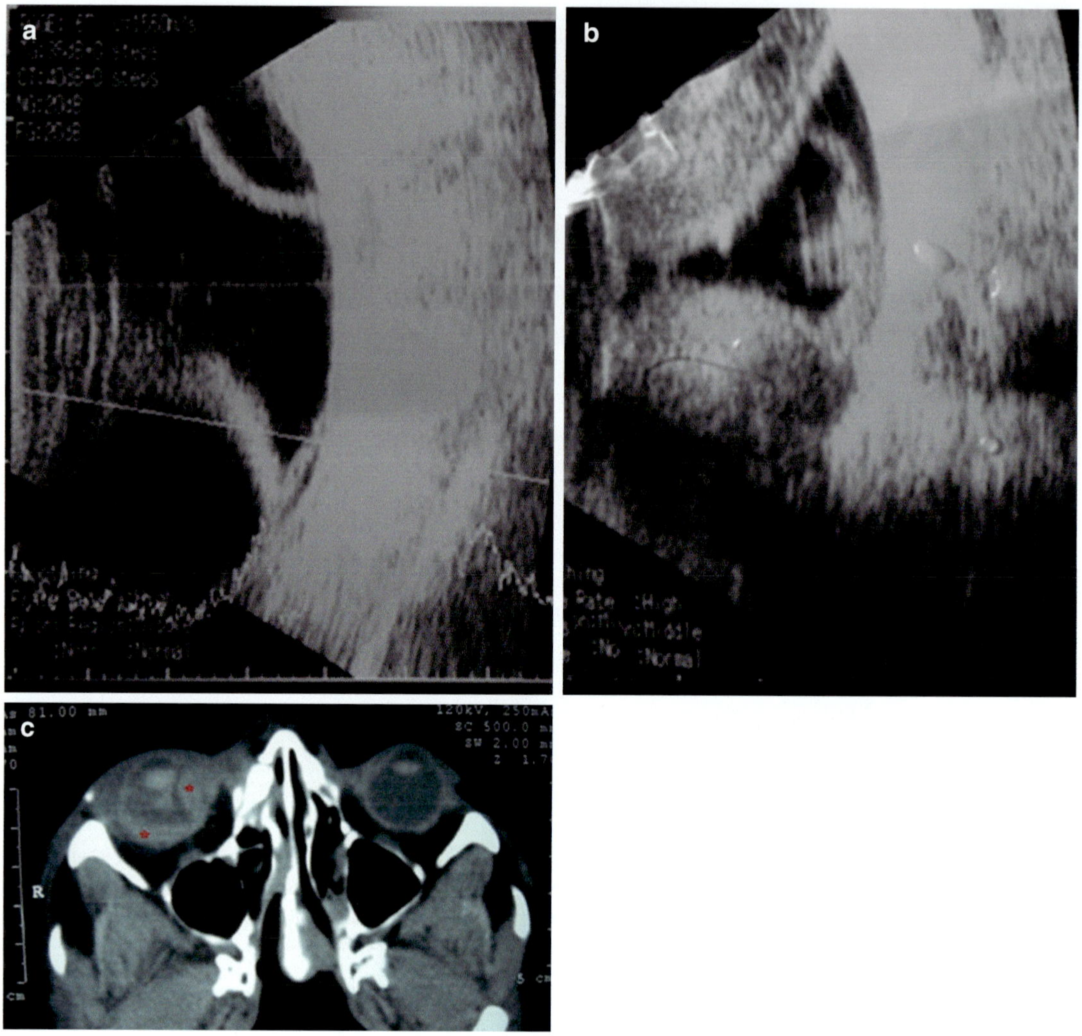

Fig. 6.7 (**a**) Serous choroidal detachment and (**b**) hemorrhagic choroidal detachment demonstrated by ocular USG. (**c**) Hemorrhagic choroidal detachment (*red stars*) demonstrated by orbital CT

subconjunctival hemorrhage is a strong indicator of ocular trauma in children and helpful especially in cases of poor cooperation (Fig. 6.8).
  - Treatment is not necessary if it is sole.
  - It may be associated with occult scleral lacerations, and in eyes with occult laceration suspicion (lower IOP, distorted pupil, vitreous hemorrhage, wrinkled lens capsule), surgical exploration is required.
- *Conjunctival laceration*:
  - Larger lacerations require saturation.
- *Corneal foreign body*:

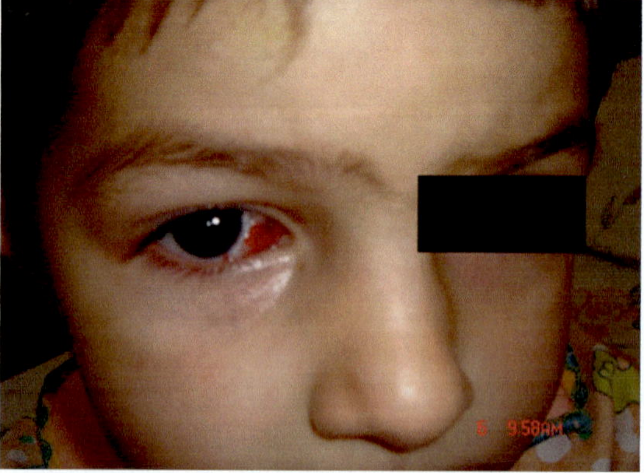

Fig. 6.8 Traumatic subconjunctival hemorrhage in a child after a needle penetrating nasal sclera

  - Superficial foreign bodies can be removed in the biomicroscope with cotton wool tips or sharp needle (Fig. 6.9).
  - Deep corneal foreign bodies (unless they are not penetrated anterior chamber) should be removed in operating room in noncompliant children.
- *Corneal erosion*:
  - Erosion is usually characterized with pain, tearing, photophobia, and decreased vision.
  - Child often keeps the eye closed.
  - Erosion is detected with fluorescein dye testing (Fig. 6.10).
- *Corneal/scleral lacerations-ruptures*:
  - Corneal laceration is the most common finding in pediatric open globe injuries [18].
  - Sports injuries and automobile crashes (airbag injuries) are major causes of globe rupture in older children [41].
  - Certain eyes are prone to rupture with minor trauma (Ehlers-Danlos syndrome, osteogenesis imperfecta) [42].
  - Ruptures occur generally in the weakest point of the eyewall (behind the insertion of the extraocular muscles).
  - Subconjunctival hemorrhage, distorted pupil, shallow anterior chamber, wrinkled lens capsule, and lowered intraocular pressure may be the signs of occult penetration.
  - The Seidel test is used to determine the leakage of aqueous humor.
    - In some self-sealing corneal wounds, gentle pressure may help to detect the leakage from the wound.
  - Bandage contact lenses may be sufficient in self-sealing partial-thickness lacerations (suturing may be necessary in noncompliant patients).
  - In cases with full-thickness laceration, prompt primary globe repair should be performed to restore the structural integrity as well as prevention of infection in children.
  - Fibrin clots often form quickly in children after primary repair and may simulate lens cortex appearance.
  - Children under the age of 9 are at risk for amblyopia. Refractive correction with spectacles or contact lens combined with occlusion therapy should start as soon as possible.
  - In adults, sutures are generally removed after 3 months. But the pediatric cornea is less rigid and sutures are loosened earlier than adults.
  - Leukoma and anterior synechiae are the common sequelae of corneal laceration [43].
  - In extensive corneal opacities, penetrating keratoplasty (PK) may be indicated.
  - In children reported rate of 1-year graft survival is between 70 and 100 %, but long-term graft survival is not so good [44–47].

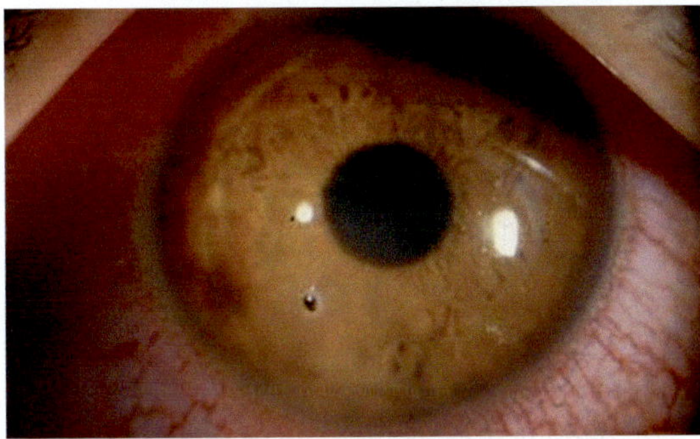

Fig. 6.9 Corneal metallic foreign body in a 16-year-old child while working at a repair industry

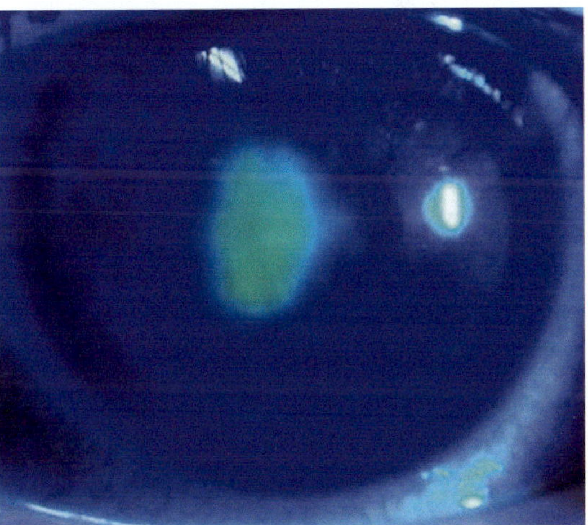

Fig. 6.10 Corneal erosion that is easily demonstrated by fluorescein dye testing and visualized by blue filter of pen light in a child that cannot be examined by slit lamp microscopy

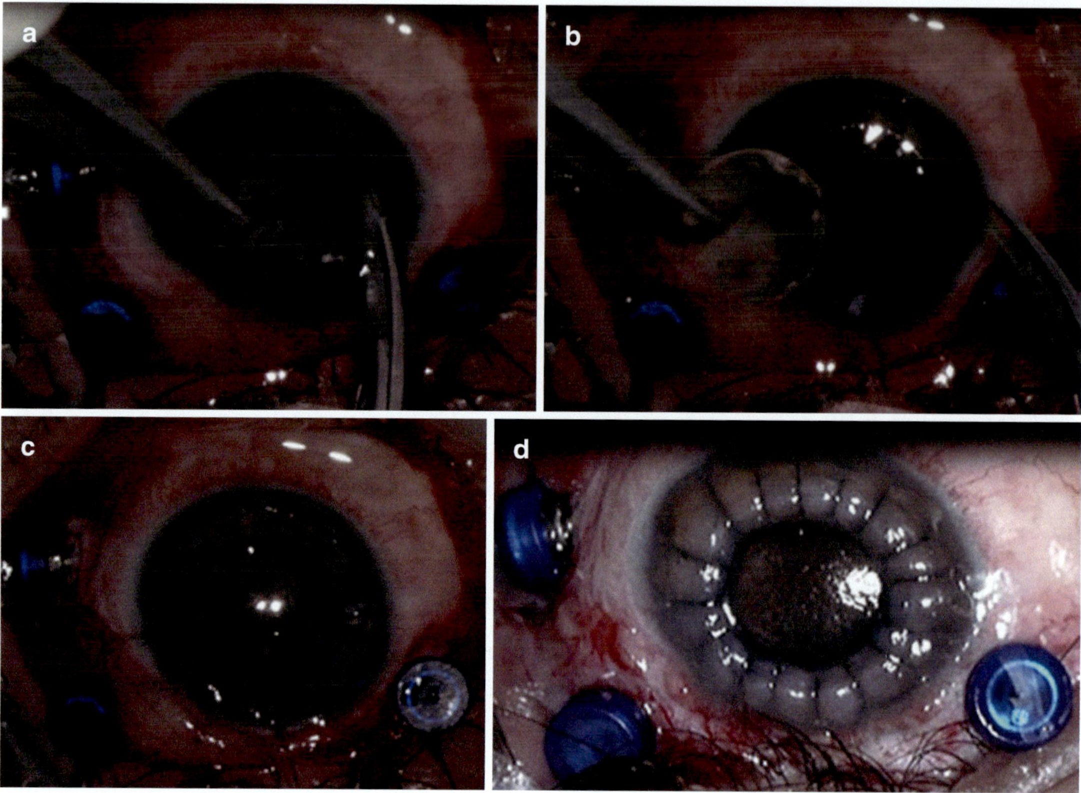

Fig. 6.11 (**a**, **b**) Removing corneal disk after trephining. (**c**) Temporary keratoprosthesis and (**d**) PK completed following posterior segment surgery

Also in cases of PK combined with vitreoretinal surgeries, prognosis is poor [48, 49].

- PK is necessary if corneal opacity is obscuring posterior segment visualization in the presence of a serious posterior segment pathology (retinal detachment, choroidal detachment, intraocular foreign body, etc.). In such cases, a temporary keratoprosthesis is used during the operation, and PK is performed at the end of the operation (Fig. 6.11a–d).
- Interrupted sutures should be used and removed earlier due to high rate of vascularization in children [50].

• *Traumatic hyphema*:
  - Hyphema occurs due to tearing of iris vessels after blunt trauma or direct insult of the eye by penetrating object (Fig. 6.12).
  - Child abuse should be considered. Furthermore, intraocular tumors (retinoblastoma) or bleeding diathesis should be kept in mind.
  - Complications are secondary hemorrhage, increased IOP, optic atrophy, peripheral anterior synechiae, and corneal staining (Fig. 6.13).
  - Children with clotting problems are prone to secondary hemorrhage.
  - Due to the difficulty of detecting early corneal blood staining and measuring the IOP in younger children, early surgical intervention may be advocated in total hyphema that persists for 4 or 5 days (Fig. 6.12).
  - Inpatient or outpatient management is controversial.
  - Parents should be warned for activity limitation, medication use, and follow-up examinations in outpatient management [51].
  - Hospitalization is indicated if parents are not able to supervise the child for strict bed

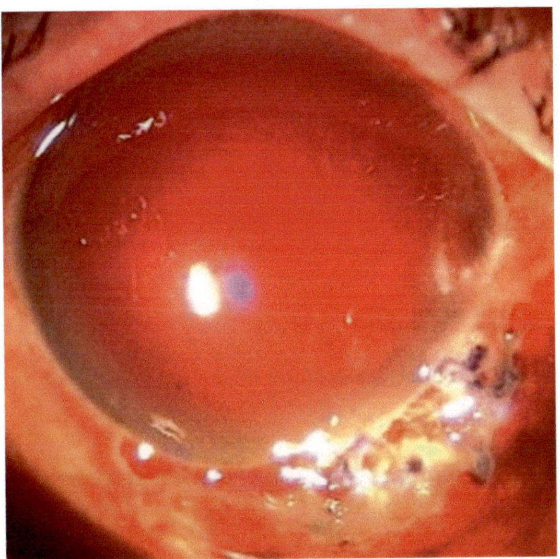

Fig. 6.12 Total hyphema with scleral rupture

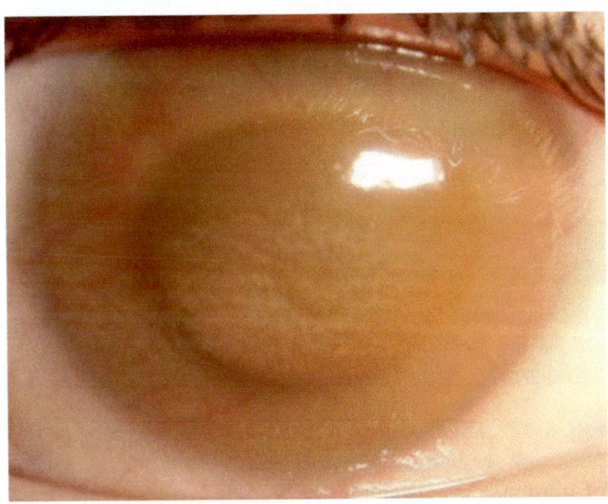

Figure 6.13 Corneal staining by hemosiderin

rest, large hyphema exists, or the child has sickle cell disease.

- *Traumatic cataract*:
  - Traumatic cataracts account for 29% of all childhood cataract and may occur after both open and closed globe injuries [52] (Fig. 6.14).
- An abnormal red reflex or leukocoria may indicate the presence of cataract in preverbal children.
  - Partial cataracts may not require surgical intervention in older children by determining visual acuity with the Snellen chart.
- *Pupil-iris problems*

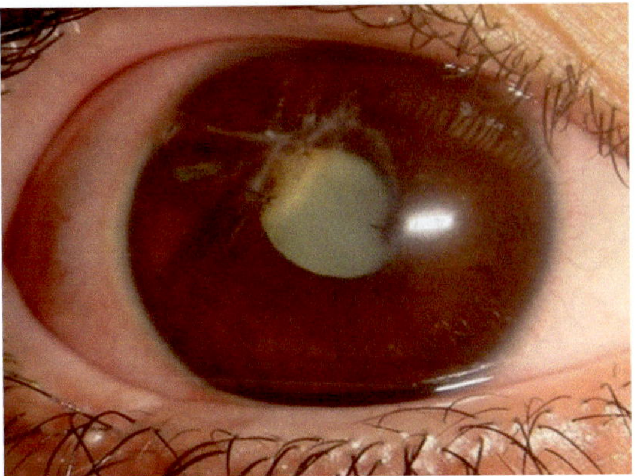

Fig. 6.14 Traumatic cataract formation in a case of open globe injury

6.4.1 Iridodialysis

Iridodialysis may result in monocular diplopia, photophobia in larger defects, and cosmetic problems. Iridodialysis can be fixed surgically (Fig. 6.15a, b).

6.4.2 Total Aniridia

Partial or total iris defects (Fig. 6.16) also cause photophobia, visual impairment, and cosmetic problems. Artificial iris implantations, aniridia contact lenses, or sclerally fixated aniridia lenses (Fig. 6.17) are frequently used treatment options.

6.5 Posterior Segment Injuries and Management

- Management of posterior segment injuries requires special attention in children due to:
  - Different anatomical structures:
    - Distance of pars plana from the limbus is closer when compared to adults so corneoscleral lacerations may be related with anterior retinal damages.
      - *Remember surgical* sclerotomy sites from the limbus:
        - <6 months: 1.5 mm
        - 6–12 months: 2 mm
        - 1–2 years: 2.5 mm
        - 2–6 years: 3 mm

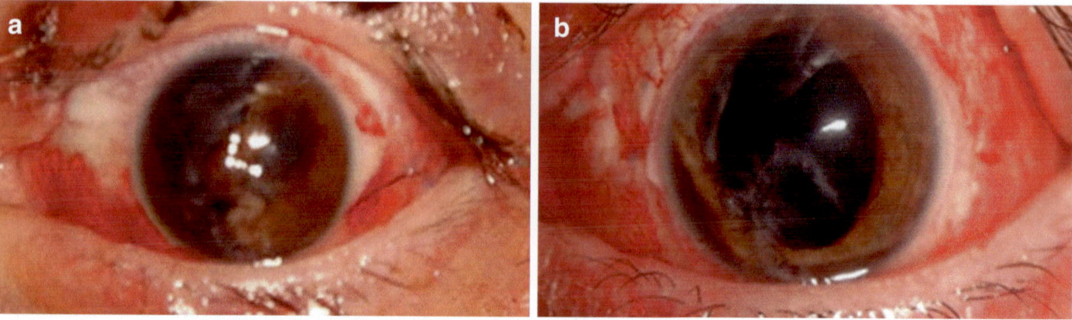

Fig. 6.15 (**a**) A 16-year-old boy: iridodialysis, traumatic cataract, and retinal detachment after a traffic accident. (**b**) Same patient after combined surgery including iridodialysis repair

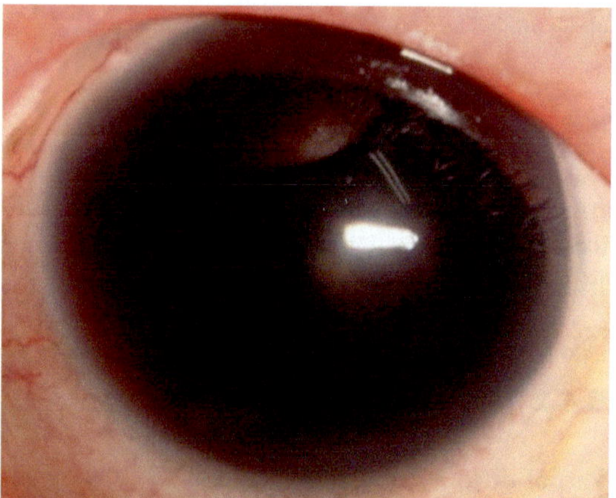

Fig. 6.16 Total traumatic aniridia

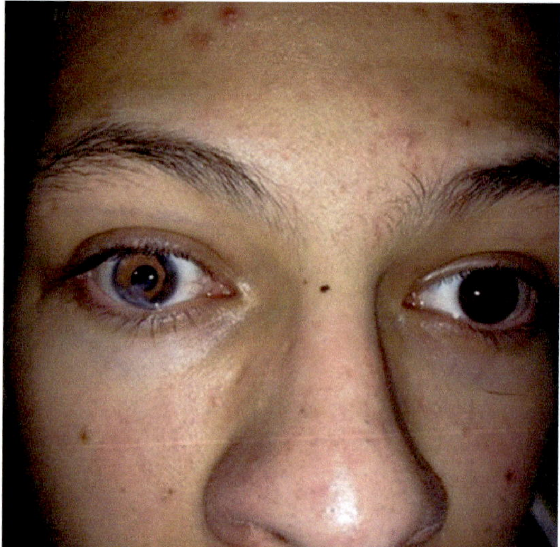

Fig. 6.17 This is another case of combined anterior and posterior segment trauma. He was 7 years old at the time of trauma. Corneoscleral penetration, total aniridia, traumatic cataract, and retinal detachment were prominent findings. After successful repair of retinal detachment, anterior segment reconstruction was done secondarily. He was complaining about photophobia. Ophtec aniridia lens was the choice for the correction of aniridia and aphakia together. This picture is 7 years after the surgery

  - Shorter axial length: Penetrating injuries may involve posterior segment structures with relatively shorter penetrations compared to adult age.
- – Increased proliferative response and scar development [15, 53]
- – More adherence of vitreous to the retina (difficulty of inducing posterior vitreous detachment (PVD) during surgery) and lens capsule
- – Amblyopia risk under age of 9 years [8].

- *Vitreous hemorrhage*:
  - – Unlike in adults (PVD or diabetic retinopathy), trauma is the main cause of vitreous hemorrhage in children (73.1 %) [54].
  - – Vitreous hemorrhage may occur after blunt or penetrating injuries, shaken baby syndrome, trivial trauma in children with blood dyscrasia, or Terson's syndrome which is exclusively related with traumatic subdural hemorrhage in children (Fig. 6.2a, b).
  - – Younger children do not complain decreased visual acuity, floaters, or pain; they present with strabismus, abnormal red reflex, or nystagmus.
  - – Vitreous hemorrhage may obscure the accompanying retinal pathologies that can

lead to retinal detachment. Furthermore, it precipitates the fibroblastic intraocular proliferation more prominently and acts as a scaffold for intraocular proliferation [55, 56].
  - Vitreous hemorrhage is a major risk factor in the development of proliferative vitreoretinopathy [57].
  - Severe vitreous hemorrhage following ocular trauma has a low rate of spontaneous clearing [58].
  - Vitrectomy should:
    - Be performed cautiously owing to strong adhesions between the vitreous and retina; otherwise, it may cause iatrogenic retinal breaks or retinal detachment [59].
      - Remove the vitreous completely to prevent posterior or anterior proliferative vitreoretinopathy [60, 61].
- *Retinal detachment*:
  - Trauma is the major cause of retinal detachment in pediatric population [62, 63].
  - Retinal detachment is characterized with late diagnosis that is associated with more frequent macula-off status, extensive multiple-quadrant retinal detachment, and higher rates of PVR development in children [62, 64–66].
  - RD occurs:
    - Due to retinal torn on the impact site.
    - Due to retinal breaks: retinal dialysis (Fig. 6.18), flap tears (Fig. 6.19), giant tears, necrotic tears, or retinal incarceration.

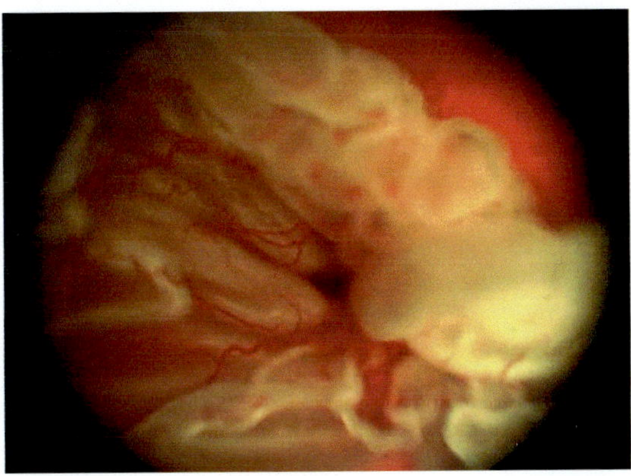

Fig. 6.18 Retinal detachment with retinal dialysis

- Commonly, initiation of an intraocular fibrocellular proliferation from the wound site through the vitreous gel and the retinal surface with membrane formation and contraction of these membranes leads to tractional retinal detachment (Fig. 6.20) [60].
  - Delayed surgical intervention and increased fibroblastic activity in children higher than adults account for high frequency of PVR development (up to 64 %) in pediatric population [64].
  - PVR is the main cause of surgical failure following RD repair (two thirds of cases) [64].
  - Surgical treatment is vitrectomy, scleral buckle, or a combination of these procedures.

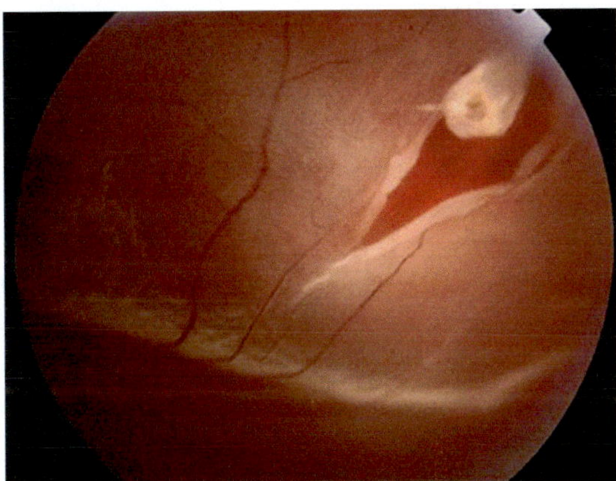

Fig. 6.19 Retinal detachment with retinal flap tears

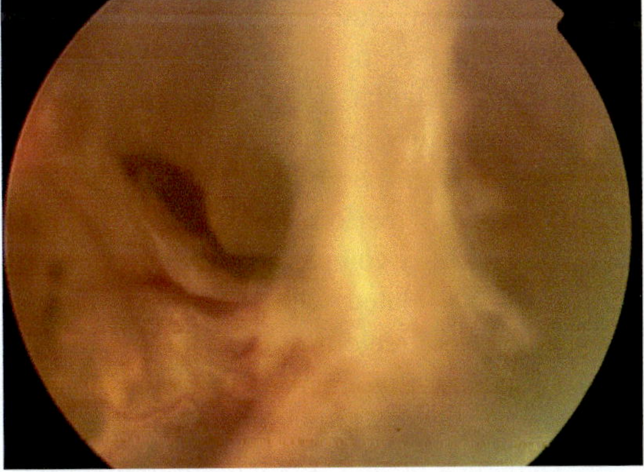

Fig. 6.20 Retinal detachment with intraocular fibrocellular proliferation

- Scleral buckle:
  - It is used to support the vitreous base and relief the anteroposterior traction.
  - Its use in children is unique aspects because:
    - Sclera is thinner and thinner suture materials should be used.
    - <2 years a 2 mm, >2 years a 2.5 mm encircling band is used.
    - Scleral buckle should be cut if the retina has stable reattachment following surgery due to complications such as extraocular muscle instability and refractive amblyopia caused by myopia.
- Vitrectomy is preferred in eyes with:
  - Rupture or perforating injuries
  - Traumatic cataract with posterior capsule injury
  - Vitreous hemorrhage
  - Tractional or hemorrhagic retinal detachment
  - Retinal incarceration
  - Giant retinal tear
  - Advanced PVR
- While performing vitrectomy, tenting of the retina indicates very strong vitreoretinal adherence [38].
- Vitrectomy should be complete to prevent proliferative vitreoretinopathy development and surgical failure [60, 61, 67].
- Visual outcomes (final visual acuity > 20/200) of traumatic retinal detachment are between 0 and 69 % [8, 15]. Poor visual outcome is associated with younger age, the presence of PVR, preoperative macular detachment, poor initial visual acuity, and eyes requiring vitrectomy [64, 68].
- Vitrectomy performed in eyes has poor visual acuity compared to scleral buckling, but it is related with the severity of the injury in vitrectomized eyes rather than the surgical technique [34].

- *Traumatic macular hole*:
  - Generally occurs after a blunt trauma [69].
  - Spontaneous closure rate is higher in children than adults (50 % vs 28 %) [70].
  - Strong vitreoretinal adhesions in children challenge to create PVD which is important for surgical success.
  - Autologous plasmin is used to facilitate PVD formation in children [71].
  - To increase closure rates, surgery is performed with TGF-beta or platelet derivates [72, 73].
  - Silicone oil may be the choice as endotamponade in noncompliant younger children.
- *Endophthalmitis*:
  - Incidence of endophthalmitis is between 0–16.5 % [74, 75].
  - In children, endophthalmitis following open globe injuries is encountered higher than adults (54.2 %) [76] (Fig. 6.21).
  - Higher incidence of traumatic endophthalmitis may be related with high rate of delay in diagnosis and treatment in children [76].
  - Causative microbial agent is different in children from adults. In children, streptococcus species and in adults staphylococcus species are the predominant microbial agents [77, 78].
  - Risk factors for endophthalmitis after open globe injury:
    - Delay in primary repair [76, 79]
    - Injury in rural setting (this was stated to show the soil contamination) [75]
    - Dirty wound [79]
    - Presence of intraocular foreign body [80]
    - Lens capsule rupture [79]

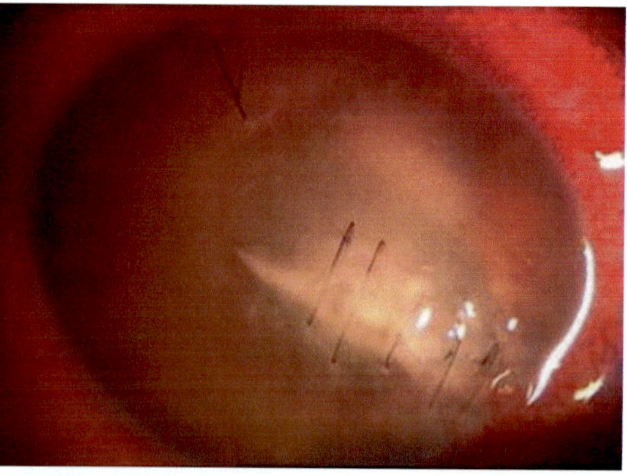

Fig. 6.21 Endophthalmitis following open globe injury

- In children, lens capsule rupture is not determined as a risk factor for posttraumatic endophthalmitis [76, 81].
- Immediate vitrectomy combined with intravitreal injection of 1 mg/0.1 mL vancomycin and 2.24 mg/0.1 mL ceftazidime is the treatment of acute posttraumatic endophthalmitis [67].
- In children, retinal detachment is encountered more than adults following endophthalmitis (57.1 % vs 8.3 %) [82, 83].

6.5.1 Current Consensuses for the Timing of Cataract Removal and IOL Implantation

In cases with anterior lens capsule tear which can cause rapid IOP elevation to high levels in children or anterior lens dislocation which can cause a pupillary block, primary lensectomy should be combined to primary wound repair in open globe injuries. In closed globe injuries, cataract extraction is generally combined with IOL implantation in children older than 2 years old at the time of trauma or hospital admission. In open globe injuries, generally, a delayed cataract extraction and primary IOL implantation are preferred after primary wound repair older than 2 years old unless posterior segment involvement is present. In combined anterior and posterior segment injuries, simultaneous cataract extraction and vitreoretinal surgery may be performed, and IOL implantation may be planned when the posterior segment, particularly the retina, is stabilized [67].

6.5.2 Management

- Treatment is surgical:
  - Anterior limbal approach:
    - Extracapsular cataract extraction or lens aspiration.
    - Anterior approach may be performed in cases with posterior capsule rupture.
  - Pars plana approach:
    - In cases with posterior capsule rupture or posteriorly dislocated lens
- Capsulorhexis is difficult to perform because anterior capsule is more elastic which may cause peripheral run.
- If posterior capsule is violated, aspiration of the lens should be performed with vitrectomy probe rather than irrigation/aspiration cannula either anterior or posterior approach.
- Intracapsular cataract extraction should not be attempted owing to strong adhesion of posterior lens capsule to anterior vitreous face.
- *IOL implantation*: Today, IOL implantation is the preferred method in correction of aphakia [84–86]. IOL provides stable optical correction, binocularity, and stereopsis and good compliance to amblyopia treatment [87, 88].
- *IOL-related complications*:
  - Fibrinous anterior uveitis:
    - Is the most early complication (as high as 81 %) [89]
    - Is prominent in dark irides [90]
  - Iris capture, synechiae, and IOL decentration [91]
  - Posterior capsule opacification (up to 100 %) [92]

6.5.3 Current Consensuses for the Choice of IOL at Different Ages

6.5.3.1 Types of IOL

Preferred IOLs are acrylic or PMMA (heparin surface modified) lenses in all age groups.

Advantages of Acrylic Lenses over PMMA Lenses

- Less postoperative complications such as PCO, fibrin, and synechiae [93, 94]:
- Greater biocompatibility.
- Smaller incision size.
- Easier implantation, adaptation, and well centration in small capsular bag [94].
- In cases without a capsular support, iris or scleral fixated IOLs may be used.
  - *Iris-fixated IOLs*:
    - Complications are retinal detachment, fibrinous uveitis, and vitreous strands into the wound [95].

  - Endothelial cell loss is significant compared to non-operated eye, but this is related with the initial corneal trauma rather than lens [95].
- *Scleral fixated IOLS*:
  - Complications are IOL dislocation due to suture breakage, vitreous hemorrhage, ocular hypertension, or hypotony [96, 97].

6.5.3.2 IOL Power

Generally, undercorrection is used for the determination of IOL power. Recommended postoperative refractions in undercorrected eyes for different age groups in different studies are:

(a) 1–2 year, +6 D; 2–4 year, +5/+3 D; 4–6 year, +3/+1 D [98]
(b) 2–3 year, +5 D; 4 year, +4 D; 5 year, +3 D [99]
(c) 1–2 year, +4 D; 3–4 year, +3 D; 5–6 year, +2 D; 7–8 year, +1 D [100]

6.5.4 Current Controversies and Alternative Management for the Timing of Cataract Extraction and IOL Implantation

Timing of cataract surgery (along with primary wound repair or a secondary intervention after primary repair) and IOL implantation (primary or secondary) are the controversial areas in traumatic cataract management. Primary IOL implantation may be performed simultaneously with primary surgical repair of open globe injuries or after a second-sitting cataract extraction. Primary cataract extraction along with primary globe repair is indicated in cases of anterior capsule rupture, anterior lens dislocations, and lens vitreous mixture.

- *Primary (immediate) cataract removal*:
  - Procedure provides control of inflammation and avoids IOP raise due to soft lens materials.
  - Procedure provides examination of the retina and optic nerve.
  - But procedure requires full equipment, instruments. and experienced staff while performing surgery.
  - Furthermore, procedure may challenge the surgeon owing to unstable wound, corneal edema, and high vitreous pressure.
- *Secondary cataract extraction*:
  - Provides complete evaluation of intraocular structures determining accompanying injuries (vitreous hemorrhage, intraocular foreign body, retinal detachment, posterior capsule rupture, etc.) after trauma.
  - Provides planning of the surgery and safest approach:
    - Adequate clear cornea
    - Formed anterior chamber
    - Good visualization of lens capsule
  - Procedure provides possibility of appropriate IOL estimation from the injured eye.
  - Requires a good control of inflammation.
- *Primary IOL implantation*:
  - Is the preferred method and has better visual outcome in many reported studies.
  - Avoids difficulties in IOL insertion into the sulcus due to posterior synechiae.
  - Provides easier IOL implantation into the capsular bag.
  - But effect of IOL on ocular growth is uncertain.
  - Furthermore, correction of aphakia with IOL may result with overcorrection due to myopic shift. A large myopic shift is encountered in children younger than 2 years old, and it may require a reoperation or contact lens fitting.
  - Postoperative inflammation may be higher than secondary IOL implantation.
  - Postoperative inflammation seems to be higher in cases with sulcus implantation compared to the bag implantations, which may be related with the contact of haptics to vascularized uveal tissue [101].
  - Has IOL-related complications:
    - *Along with primary wound repair*:
      - Procedure avoids additional surgery, use of anesthetics, time, and cost.
      - Procedure provides faster and better visual rehabilitation consequently

prevention of amblyopia. Therefore, one-step surgery (primary wound repair + primary cataract extraction + IOL implantation) may be advocated in younger children.
  - Procedure has a higher risk of endophthalmitis.
  - Furthermore, visualization of posterior segment during examination or surgical intervention may be limited due to pupil distortion.
  - In this procedure, IOL power cannot be estimated in a fresh injured eye. The fellow eye is used for IOL power calculation. However, high deviation from the predicted refraction may occur.
- *Along with secondary cataract extraction*:
  - Is the most administered method in many studies and has satisfactory visual results.
  - Has the advantage of performing implantation in a quite eye.
  - Refractive power of the IOL can be performed from the injured eye.
  - Therefore, IOL power estimation may be more predictable.
  - Should be performed as soon as possible in young children because interval between trauma and surgery has a prognostic value.
- *Secondary IOL implantation*:
  - Provides planning the surgery in a quite eye.
  - Provides information about the potential visual outcome.
  - Provides an accurate IOL power estimation.
  - In cases with posterior segment involvement, secondary implantation may be more appropriate for both visualization and surgical intervention of the peripheral retina. Furthermore, IOL power may change due to vitreoretinal surgeries.
  - IOL is usually inserted to sulcus due to fusion of anterior and posterior capsule leaves.
  - Posterior synechiolysis may be necessary before inserting IOL to sulcus.
  - But, visual outcome seems to be poor compared to primary IOL implantation.

6.5.5 Proposed Methods for Correction of Aphakia Other than IOL Implantation

- *Spectacles*: not preferable for unilateral cases.
- *Contact lenses*:
- Contact lens wear may be suggested for children younger than 2 years old particularly in infants due to existence of unpredictability of postoperative refraction and higher rates of IOL complications [89, 102]. Although visual outcomes and binocularity are inferior compared to IOL implantation, postoperative complications such as visual axis opacification, inflammation, and reoperations for complications are lower than IOL implantation [87, 91, 92, 103–105]. Also, compliance of contact lens wear is better in younger children.

IOL implantation may be performed after 2 years old when the increase at axial length gets slower [106]. Furthermore, in high astigmatic corneas due to scar formation, contact lenses may be fitted for astigmatic correction in IOL-implanted eyes. Drawbacks of contact lens wear are difficulty in inserting or removing lens, infection, loss of lens, high cost due to frequent change for refractive correction, and difficulty in compliance.

Contact lens implementation has less favorable results due to high cost and noncompliance particularly in children older than 2 years old and lower visual outcome despite immediate correction and patching [92].

For the correction of aphakia combined with iris defects, contact lenses may be preferable (Fig. 6.22a, b).

When there is high or irregular astigmatism arising from corneal surface, contact lenses may still be the best option for refractive correction for the elderly children.

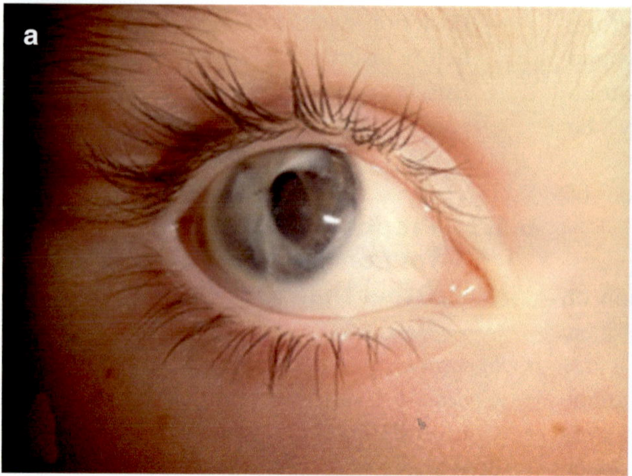

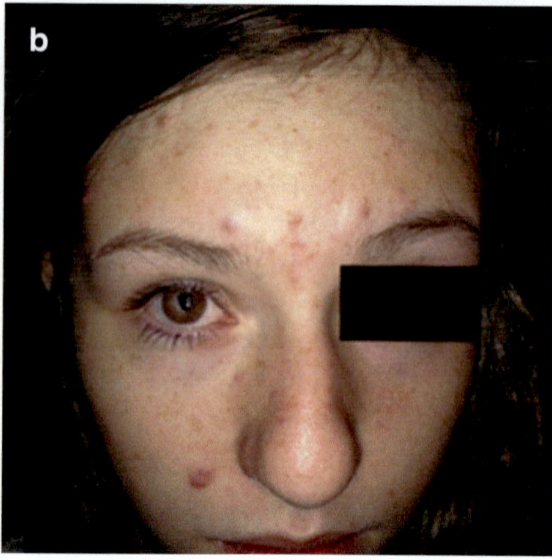

Fig. 6.22 (**a**, **b**) This is a case of combined anterior and posterior segment trauma. She was 5 years old at the time of trauma. Corneoscleral penetration, partial aniridia, traumatic cataract, vitreous hemorrhage, and retinal detachment were prominent findings. After successful repair, she was wearing aphakic contact lenses for refractive errors. She is now 13 years old, and a color contact lens is recommended (**b**) in order to cover corneal scar (**a**) tissue for cosmetic aims

6.5.6 Current Controversies for the Choice of IOL for Children at Different Ages

Calculating the appropriate IOL power for optimized refractive and visual outcome in children is a unique problem. This problem arises from the unpredictability of axial elongation in children and estimation errors of IOL formulas. The amount of axial elongation is influenced by inheritance, cataract, and age of child [107–109]. Axial elongation is rapid in the first 2 years of life and continues in a slow manner until the first decade [106]. In other words, myopic shift following IOL implantation is related with the amount of axial elongation, and generally large myopic shifts occur in younger children [110–113]. O'Keefe et al. [110] found a −6 D myopic shift in the first 24 months, Dahan and Drusedau [111] −6.39 D in 12–18 months, and Crouch et al. [112] −5.69 D in 12–24 months and −3.66 D after 3 years old. McClatchey et al. [113] found a total of 6.6 D myopic shift in 11 years and determined greater myopic shift and variability in predictive refractive change younger than 2 years old. Furthermore, most of the IOL formulas are developed for adult eyes and may lead to refractive prediction errors owing to shorter axial lengths and steeper corneas in younger children particularly in age less than 2 years old. SRK II, SRK T, Hoffer Q, and Holladay 1 are the preferred formulas in determining IOL power in pediatric cataracts. But in shorter eyes (axial length < 22 mm), Hoffer Q seems to be the most predictable formula.

Undercorrection of IOL power due to the age of the child is implemented for providing the child to become emmetropic or mild ametropic in the later life. In other words children are expected to have less spectacle or contact lens dependent and better stereopsis.

On the other hand, some clinicians favor an IOL implantation that targets an emmetropic postoperative refraction. Some pseudophakic eyes may encounter minimal myopic shift or may have smaller axial elongation than unoperated fellow eye [114, 115]. In other words, it is concluded that prediction of the effect of IOL on axial length or myopic shift accurately is difficult in growing eyes. Furthermore, with emmetropization, children would have better near and mid-distance vision without the need of correction that can avoid amblyopia development.

The most controversial age group in IOL implantation is infants. Although visual outcome and binocularity are better in pseudophakic eyes compared to aphakic eyes, unpredicted large myopic shift, higher intraocular inflammation, visual axis opacification (secondary membranes at anterior or posterior of IOL), insignificant rate of glaucoma compared to aphakia, and high rate of additional surgeries (IOL exchange for large myopic shift, membranectomy for visual axis opacification) are the drawbacks of IOL implantation in infants [116].

6.5.7 Primary or Secondary Posterior Capsulotomy After IOL Implantation

In-the-bag IOL implantation is the preferred technique because contact of IOL with uveal tissue is minimized, and consequently postoperative inflammation and IOL decentration are low. Nevertheless, PCO rate is higher in traumatic cases due to inflammation owing to nature of the trauma. Incidence can be as high as 100 % [92]. PCO is a vision-threatening complication following IOL implantation in children. Because clear visual axis is the mainstay of prevention of amblyopia development, there have been several methods to clear visual axis.

YAG laser capsulotomy:

- Is a secondary procedure.
- Is a noninvasive method.
- Can provide a clear visual axis in early days.
- Re-opacification usually occurs particularly in younger children [117, 118].

Primary posterior capsulorhexis with optic capture:

- Is recommended for preventing secondary opacification and obtains better optic centration [119].
- However, secondary opacification may be encountered [120].
- Furthermore, IOL exchange is difficult later.

Primary posterior capsulotomy with anterior vitrectomy:

- Is recommended for children less than 10 years old and for those who will not follow their control examinations [85, 90].
- Anterior vitrectomy is combined to primary posterior capsulotomy due to re-opacification on anterior hyaloid face [121].
- Re-opacification rate is lower [122, 123].

6.5.8 Current Consensuses for the Timing of Vitrectomy

In general, simultaneous vitreoretinal intervention and primary globe repair are suggested for injuries with IOFB and endophthalmitis [12]. In other cases, most of the surgeons prefer performing vitrectomy after 4 days and before 2 weeks to make easier surgery for two reasons: adequate PVD formation which is important for complete vitreous removal and reduced intraocular congestion which may be related with reduced intraocular hemorrhage during intervention. Several studies have demonstrated good visual outcomes with this approach [8, 124].

6.5.8.1 Current Controversies and Alternative Managements for the Timing of Vitrectomy

Vitrectomy is widely used in the treatment of traumatic retinal detachments, perforating injuries, intraocular foreign bodies, and endophthalmitis. In eyes with dense vitreous hemorrhage and attached retina, performing surgery or observation is controversial due to lack of evidence-based studies. However, observation of vitreous hemorrhage in children carries the risk of PVR and amblyopia development. Severe vitreous hemorrhage is associated with a slow clearance rate, and particularly younger children are prone to develop a pronounced proliferative response [58]. In the experimental animal models, only the eyes which were injected with autologous blood showed marked intraocular proliferation and total tractional retinal detachment [55, 125]. In another animal model, eyes which underwent vitrectomy had a markedly decreased rate of tractional retinal detachment. In other words, vitrectomy not only clears the visual axis but also prevents the development of PVR by clearing the stimulus and scaffold for intraocular proliferation [60]. Furthermore, vitrectomy exposes and gives chance to detect and treat the retinal pathologies beneath the hemorrhage. However, timing of vitrectomy is still controversial. Vitrectomy may be performed simultaneously with primary globe repair or may be delayed for a while (within 3 days, 4–14 days and after 2 weeks).

6.5.9 Simultaneous Primary Globe Repair and Vitrectomy

This option requires an experienced vitreoretinal surgeon performing the whole procedure or near for consultation and completing the internal reconstruction.

- Advantages:
  - Decreased risk of endophthalmitis
  - Decreased rate of inflammatory reaction and PVR
  - Prevention of retinal detachment development
  - Prevention of secondary ciliary body damage
- Disadvantages:
  - Difficulty due to central corneal wound or corneal edema
  - Risk of expulsive choroidal hemorrhage
  - Hypotony due to wound leak
  - Difficulty in surgery due to incomplete PVD
  - Difficulty in preparing the surgical equipment and personnel
  - Difficulty in planning the whole management strategy due to limited time

6.5.10 Delayed Internal Reconstruction

- *Within 3 days*:
  - This approach was originally proposed by Coleman. It offers the most advantages of primary simultaneous surgery except decrease in endophthalmitis risk.
  - With the utilization of steroid treatment immediately after primary repair, the risk of expulsive hemorrhage is reduced.
- *4–14 days*:
  - This is the widely accepted approach.
  - Advantages:
    - Facility in planning the whole management
    - Lower risk of expulsive choroidal hemorrhage with steroid treatment
    - Facility in performing surgery due to the presence of adequate posterior vitreous detachment
    - Facility in intraoperative hemorrhage control
    - Facility in clearing hemorrhagic retinal and choroidal detachments due to liquefied cloth
    - Prepared surgical equipment and personnel
  - Disadvantages:
    - Probability of retinal detachment existence and initiated PVR
- *After 2 weeks*:
  - Advantages:
    - Surgery can be performed easily due to spontaneous separation of posterior hyaloid.
    - Allows liquefaction of choroidal hemorrhage and enables removing hemorrhage.
  - Disadvantages:
    - Existence of retinal detachment and pronounced PVR

In other cases, vitreoretinal intervention is being performed after primary globe repair. Open globe injuries with vitreous hemorrhage are associated with intraocular proliferation and ultimately with tractional retinal detachment [55, 125]. This proliferative response is pronounced in children. Intraocular proliferation starts with as early as 4 days after injury and proponents of vitrectomy within the first 72 h state that vitrectomy avoids formation and recurrence of this intraocular proliferation [126]. Proponents of this approach determined that visual outcomes of this approach were better than the patients operated at a later time.

In experimental animal models, vitrectomy was performed on day 1 and day 14, and there was no significant difference among them in terms of prevention of intraocular proliferation and retinal detachment [56, 60]. Furthermore, in day 1, peripheral vitreous cleaning was more difficult due to inadequate PVD formation which is more prominent in children owing to strong vitreoretinal adhesions. Peripheral and base vitreous cleaning (complete vitrectomy) is easy with adequate PVD and necessary to prevent anterior and posterior reproliferation [60]. Therefore, most of the surgeons prefer performing vitrectomy after 4 days and before 2 weeks to make easier surgery for two reasons: adequate PVD formation which is important for complete vitreous removal and reduced intraocular congestion which may be related with reduced intraocular hemorrhage during intervention. Several studies have demonstrated good visual outcomes with this approach [8, 124].

In a recent study by Sandinha et al., vitrectomy was performed at a mean 49 days after primary globe repair in younger patients. They have performed vitrectomy after PVD development. They did not encounter any retinal detachment and PVR with their wait-and-watch strategy [127]. Allowing formation of spontaneous PVD and recovering the eye from commotio retinae and necrosis may be an option in the reconstruction following open globe injuries. They have concluded that risk of PVR and RD development may be too overestimated. Hermsen et al. and Vatne and Syrdalen have obtained improved visual results with vitrectomy after 2 weeks [128, 129]. Furthermore, in some published studies, visual outcome was related with the extent of injury rather than the time of vitreoretinal interventions [130, 131].

Although there is no consensus in the literature about the timing of vitrectomy, children differ from adults in terms of amblyopia risk and exaggerated fibrovascular proliferation and scarring. Also a dense vitreous hemorrhage may obscure retinal tears, retinal detachment, and associated chorioretinal pathologies. Therefore, a wait-and-watch approach following ocular trauma involving posterior segment may not be prevailed in children. Early vitrectomy within 2 weeks may be the optimum approach in children. Although it is not widely used today, ocriplasmin may be used to facilitate creation of posterior vitreous detachment before surgery [132].

6.5.11 Current Consensuses for the Prevention of Amblyopia After Trauma

- Amblyopia is the main cause of low visual outcome in children less than 9 years old [9].
- Delay in referral is another cause of low visual outcome.

Amblyopia is the major concern following ocular trauma in children up to 9 years old. The main strategy in prevention of amblyopia is a prompt approach to ocular damage causing visual deprivation. Early screening following ocular trauma treatment may detect significant refractive errors and strabismus that cause anisometropic and strabismic amblyopia. In cases with aphakia, primary or secondary IOL implantation is the preferred method for a continuous refractive power [90]. Aphakic contact lenses may be an option in children up to 2 years owing to possible complications of IOL implantation. In cases with posterior segment involvement, surgical intervention within 2 weeks is stated as the optimum time of reconstruction for prevention of deprivation amblyopia [8]. Silicone oil causes approximately +5 and +6 hyperopia that can cause anisometropic amblyopia unless it is corrected. After the surgical intervention of trauma, optical correction and a vigorous occlusion therapy with a tight follow-up are the ultimate approach for the prevention of amblyopia.

Refractive error differences between traumatic and fellow eye for myopia −3 D or more, hyperopia +1 D or more, and astigmatism 1.5 D or more may cause anisometropic amblyopia. Optical correction can be utilized by spectacles and contact lenses. Although spectacles are more economic and have a protective effect on both eyes, they may cause confusion and be a barrier to binocular vision improvement. Contact lenses reduce aniseikonia, prismatic imbalance, and distortion. In children younger than 2 years old, correction of aphakia with contact lenses may be an option due to complications of IOL implantation. Contact lenses can also be utilized in silicone oil-filled eyes for correction of hyperopia. Furthermore, significant astigmatism caused by corneal scar can be corrected with rigid gas permeable contact lenses.

Amblyopia treatment must start just after the trauma surgery. Meticulous amblyopia treatment and follow-up is necessary along with surgeries and refractive correction.

Clinical Pearls for Treatment

- Corneal sutures cause corneal vascularization and scarring in children more than adults. Therefore, sutures must be removed earlier in pediatric cases.
- Sickle cell disease may cause optic atrophy at lower IOP risings and necessitate early surgical removal of hyphema.
- In pediatric traumatic macular holes, early surgical intervention may be preferable owing to high closure rate with surgery compared to spontaneous closure.
- Unless the posterior capsule rupture is present, simple aspiration of the lens may be adequate because the lens nucleus is generally soft in children.
- Primary cataract removal may prevent development of further retinal damage and proliferative vitreoretinopathy in cases with vitreous lens mixture.

References

1. Strahlman E, Elman M, Daub E, Baker S. Causes of pediatric eye injuries. A population-based study. Arch Ophthalmol (Chicago, Ill: 1960). 1990;108(4):603–6.
2. May DR, Kuhn FP, Morris RE, et al. The epidemiology of serious eye injuries from the United States Eye Injury Registry. Graefes Arch Clin Exp Ophthalmol (Albrecht von Graefes Archiv fur klinische und experimentelle Ophthalmologie). 2000;238(2):153–7.
3. Sherwin JC, Dean WH, Metcalfe N. Screening for childhood blindness and visual impairment in a secondary school in rural Malawi. Eye (London, England). 2011;25(2):256–7.
4. Salvin JH. Systemic approach to pediatric ocular trauma. Curr Opin Ophthalmol. 2007;18:366–72.
5. Khatry SK, Lewis AE, Schein OD, Thapa MD, Pradhan EK, Katz J. The epidemiology of ocular trauma in rural Nepal. Br J Ophthalmol. 2004;88(4):456–60.
6. MacEwen CJ, Baines PS, Desai P. Eye injuries in children: the current picture. Br J Ophthalmol. 1999;83(8):933–6.
7. Karaman K, Znaor L, Lakos V, Olujic I. Epidemiology of pediatric eye injury in Split-Dalmatia County. Ophthalmic Res. 2009;42(4):199–204.
8. Jandeck C, Kellner U, Bornfeld N, Foerster MH. Open globe injuries in children. Graefes Arch Clin Exp Ophthalmol (Albrecht von Graefes Archiv fur klinische und experimentelle Ophthalmologie). 2000;238(5):420–6.
9. Olitsky SE, Nelson BA, Brooks S. The sensitive period of visual development in humans. J Pediatr Ophthalmol Strabismus. 2002;39(2):69–72; quiz 105–6.
10. Podbielski DW, Surkont M, Tehrani NN, Ratnapalan S. Pediatric eye injuries in a Canadian emergency department. Can J Ophthalmol (Journal canadien d'ophtalmologie). 2009;44(5):519–22.
11. Grieshaber MC, Stegmann R. Penetrating eye injuries in South African children: aetiology and visual outcome. Eye (London, England). 2006;20(7):789–95.
12. Sul S, Gurelik G, Korkmaz S, Ozdek S, Hasanreisoglu B. Pediatric open-globe injuries: clinical characteristics and factors associated with poor visual and anatomical success. Graefes Arch Clin Exp Ophthalmol (Albrecht von Graefes Archiv fur klinische und experimentelle Ophthalmologie). 2015;254(7):1405–10.
13. Serrano JC, Chalela P, Arias JD. Epidemiology of childhood ocular trauma in a northeastern Colombian region. Arch Ophthalmol (Chicago, Ill: 1960). 2003;121(10):1439–45.
14. Rapoport I, Romem M, Kinek M, et al. Eye injuries in children in Israel. A nationwide collaborative study. Arch Ophthalmol (Chicago, Ill: 1960). 1990;108(3):376–9.
15. Moisseiev J, Vidne O, Treister G. Vitrectomy and silicone oil injection in pediatric patients. Retina (Philadelphia, PA). 1998;18(3):221–7.
16. Scharf J, Zonis S. Perforating injuries of the eye in childhood. J Pediatr Ophthalmol. 1975;13:326–8.
17. Mayouego Kouam J, Epee E, Azria S, et al. Epidemiological, clinical and therapeutic features of pediatric ocular injuries in an eye emergency unit in Ile-de-France. J Fr Ophtalmol. 2015;38(8):743–51.
18. Liu ML, Chang YS, Tseng SH, et al. Major pediatric ocular trauma in Taiwan. J Pediatr Ophthalmol Strabismus. 2010;47(2):88–95.

19. Mela EK, Georgakopoulos CD, Georgalis A, Koliopoulos JX, Gartaganis SP. Severe ocular injuries in Greek children. Ophthalmic Epidemiol. 2003;10(1):23–9.
20. Listman DA. Paintball injuries in children: more than meets the eye. Pediatrics. 2004;113(1 Pt 1):e15–8.
21. Sternberg Jr P, de Juan Jr E, Green WR, Hirst LW, Sommer A. Ocular BB injuries. Ophthalmology. 1984;91(10):1269–77.
22. Jing Y, Yi-qiao X, Yan-ning Y, Ming A, An-huai Y, Lian-hong Z. Clinical analysis of firework-related ocular injuries during Spring Festival 2009. Graefes Arch Clin Exp Ophthalmol (Albrecht von Graefes Archiv fur klinische und experimentelle Ophthalmologie). 2010;248(3):333–8.
23. Erickson BP, Cavuoto K, Rachitskaya A. Zone 3 ruptured globe from a dog bite. J AAPOS (The Official Publication of the American Association for Pediatric Ophthalmology and Strabismus/American Association for Pediatric Ophthalmology and Strabismus). 2015;19(1):89–90.
24. Lekse Kovach J, Maguluri S, Recchia FM. Subclinical endophthalmitis following a rooster attack. J AAPOS (The Official publication of the American Association for Pediatric Ophthalmology and Strabismus/ American Association for Pediatric Ophthalmology and Strabismus). 2006;10(6):579–80.
25. Yildirim N, Kabadere E, Ermis Z. Perforating corneal injury with a fish hook. Ophthalmic Surg Lasers iImaging (The Official Journal of the International Society for Imaging in the Eye). 2008;39(2):137–9.
26. Rishi E, Rishi P, Koundanya VV, Sahu C, Roy R, Bhende PS. Post-traumatic endophthalmitis in 143 eyes of children and adolescents from India. Eye (London, England). 2016;30(4):615–20.
27. Eagling EM. Perforating injuries involving the posterior segment. Trans Ophthalmol Soc U K. 1975;95(2):335–9.
28. De Juan Jr E, Sternberg Jr P, Michels RG. Penetrating ocular injuries. Types of injuries and visual results. Ophthalmology. 1983;90(11):1318–22.
29. LaRoche GR, McIntyre L, Schertzer RM. Epidemiology of severe eye injuries in childhood. Ophthalmology. 1988;95(12):1603–7.
30. Patel BC. Penetrating eye injuries. Arch Dis Child. 1989;64(3):317–20.
31. Spiegel D, Nasemann J, Nawrocki J, Gabel VP. Severe ocular trauma managed with primary pars plana vitrectomy and silicone oil. Retina (Philadelphia, PA). 1997;17(4):275–85.
32. Cao H, Li L, Zhang M, Li H. Epidemiology of pediatric ocular trauma in the Chaoshan Region, China, 2001–2010. PLoS One. 2013;8(4):e60844.
33. Pieramici DJ, Sternberg Jr P, Aaberg Sr TM, et al. A system for classifying mechanical injuries of the eye (globe). The Ocular Trauma Classification Group. Am J Ophthalmol. 1997;123(6):820–31.
34. Sheard RM, Mireskandari K, Ezra E, Sullivan PM. Vitreoretinal surgery after childhood ocular trauma. Eye (London, England). 2007;21(6):793–8.
35. Saunte JP, Saunte ME. Childhood ocular trauma in the Copenhagen area from 1998 to 2003: eye injuries caused by airsoft guns are twice as common as firework-related injuries. Acta Ophthalmol. 2008;86(3):345–7.
36. Alfaro III DV, Liggett PE. Vitreoretinal surgery of the injured eye. Philadelphia: Lippincott-Raven; 1999.
37. Hill JR, Crawford BD, Lee H, Tawansy KA. Evaluation of open globe injuries of children in the last 12 years. Retina (Philadelphia, PA). 2006;26(7 Suppl):S65–8.
38. Kuhn F. Ocular traumatology. Berlin/New York: Springer; 2008.
39. Stryjewski TP, Andreoli CM, Eliott D. Retinal detachment after open globe injury. Ophthalmology. 2014;121(1):327–33.
40. Thakker MM, Ray S. Vision-limiting complications in open-globe injuries. Can J Ophthalmol (Journal canadien d'ophtalmologie). 2006;41(1):86–92.
41. Kennedy EA, Ng TP, McNally C, Stitzel JD, Duma SM. Risk functions for human and porcine eye rupture based on projectile characteristics of blunt objects. Stapp Car Crash J. 2006;50:651–71.
42. Hoyt CS, Taylor D. Pediatric ophthalmology and strabismus. St. Louis: Elsevier; 2013.
43. Ariturk N, Sahin M, Oge I, Erkan D, Sullu Y. The evaluation of ocular trauma in children between ages 0–12. Turk J Pediatr. 1999;41(1):43–52.
44. Stulting RD, Sumers KD, Cavanagh HD, Waring 3rd GO, Gammon JA. Penetrating keratoplasty in children. Ophthalmology. 1984;91(10):1222–30.
45. Cowden JW. Penetrating keratoplasty in infants and children. Ophthalmology. 1990;97(3):324–8; discussion 8–9.
46. Dana MR, Schaumberg DA, Moyes AL, et al. Outcome of penetrating keratoplasty after ocular trauma in children. Arch Ophthalmol (Chicago, IL: 1960). 1995;113(12):1503–7.
47. Patel HY, Ormonde S, Brookes NH, Moffatt LS, McGhee CN. The indications and outcome of paediatric corneal transplantation in New Zealand: 1991–2003. Br J Ophthalmol. 2005;89(4):404–8.
48. Garcia-Valenzuela E, Blair NP, Shapiro MJ, et al. Outcome of vitreoretinal surgery and penetrating keratoplasty using temporary keratoprosthesis. Retina (Philadelphia, PA). 1999;19(5):424–9.
49. Roters S, Szurman P, Hermes S, Thumann G, Bartz-Schmidt KU, Kirchhof B. Outcome of combined penetrating keratoplasty with vitreoretinal surgery for management of severe ocular injuries. Retina (Philadelphia, PA). 2003;23(1):48–56.
50. Vajpayee RB, Angra SK, Honavar SG. Combined keratoplasty, cataract extraction, and intraocular lens implantation after corneolenticular laceration in children. Am J Ophthalmol. 1994;117(4):507–11.
51. Rocha KM, Martins EN, Melo Jr LA, Moraes NS. Outpatient management of traumatic hyphema in children: prospective evaluation. J AAPOS (The Official Publication of the American Association for Pediatric Ophthalmology and Strabismus/American

Association for Pediatric Ophthalmology and Strabismus). 2004;8(4):357–61.
52. Eckstein M, Vijayalakshmi P, Killedar M, Gilbert C, Foster A. Aetiology of childhood cataract in south India. Br J Ophthalmol. 1996;80(7):628–32.
53. Scott IU, Flynn Jr HW, Azen SP, Lai MY, Schwartz S, Trese MT. Silicone oil in the repair of pediatric complex retinal detachments: a prospective, observational, multicenter study. Ophthalmology. 1999;106(7):1399–407; discussion 407–8.
54. Spirn MJ, Lynn MJ, Hubbard 3rd GB. Vitreous hemorrhage in children. Ophthalmology. 2006;113(5):848–52.
55. Cleary PE, Ryan SJ. Histology of wound, vitreous, and retina in experimental posterior penetrating eye injury in the rhesus monkey. Am J Ophthalmol. 1979;88(2):221–31.
56. Cleary PE, Ryan SJ. Experimental posterior penetrating eye injury in the rabbit. II. Histology of wound, vitreous, and retina. Br J Ophthalmol. 1979;63(5):312–21.
57. Feng K, Hu Y, Wang C, et al. Risk factors, anatomical, and visual outcomes of injured eyes with proliferative vitreoretinopathy: eye injury vitrectomy study. Retina (Philadelphia, PA). 2013;33(8):1512–8.
58. Spraul CW, Grossniklaus HE. Vitreous Hemorrhage. Surv Ophthalmol. 1997;42(1):3–39.
59. Sebag J. Age-related differences in the human vitreoretinal interface. Arch Ophthalmol (Chicago, IL: 1960). 1991;109(7):966–71.
60. Cleary PE, Ryan SJ. Vitrectomy in penetrating eye injury. Results of a controlled trial of vitrectomy in an experimental posterior penetrating eye injury in the rhesus monkey. Arch Ophthalmol (Chicago, IL: 1960). 1981;99(2):287–92.
61. Gregor Z, Ryan SJ. Complete and core vitrectomies in the treatment of experimental posterior penetrating eye injury in the rhesus monkey. II. Histologic features. Arch Ophthalmol (Chicago, IL: 1960). 1983;101(3):446–50.
62. Soheilian M, Ramezani A, Malihi M, et al. Clinical features and surgical outcomes of pediatric rhegmatogenous retinal detachment. Retina (Philadelphia, PA). 2009;29(4):545–51.
63. Rosner M, Treister G, Belkin M. Epidemiology of retinal detachment in childhood and adolescence. J Pediatr Ophthalmol Strabismus. 1987;24(1):42–4.
64. Wang NK, Chen YP, Yeung L, et al. Traumatic pediatric retinal detachment following open globe injury. Ophthalmologica (Journal international d'ophtalmologie International journal of ophthalmology Zeitschrift fur Augenheilkunde). 2007;221(4):255–63.
65. Fivgas GD, Capone Jr A. Pediatric rhegmatogenous retinal detachment. Retina (Philadelphia, PA). 2001;21(2):101–6.
66. Guillaume JB, Godde-Jolly D, Haut J, Monin C, Ruellan YM. Surgical treatment of traumatic retinal detachment in children under 15 years of age. J Fr Ophtalmol. 1991;14(5):311–9.
67. Meier P. Combined anterior and posterior segment injuries in children: a review. Graefes Arch Clin Exp Ophthalmol (Albrecht von Graefes Archiv fur klinische und experimentelle Ophthalmologie). 2010;248(9):1207–19.
68. Sarrazin L, Averbukh E, Halpert M, Hemo I, Rumelt S. Traumatic pediatric retinal detachment: a comparison between open and closed globe injuries. Am J Ophthalmol. 2004;137(6):1042–9.
69. Johnson RN, McDonald HR, Lewis H, et al. Traumatic macular hole: observations, pathogenesis, and results of vitrectomy surgery. Ophthalmology. 2001;108(5):853–7.
70. Miller JB, Yonekawa Y, Eliott D, et al. Long-term follow-up and outcomes in traumatic macular holes. Am J Ophthalmol. 2015;160(6):1255–8.e1.
71. Wu WC, Drenser KA, Trese MT, Williams GA, Capone A. Pediatric traumatic macular hole: results of autologous plasmin enzyme-assisted vitrectomy. Am J Ophthalmol. 2007;144(5):668–72.
72. Rubin JS, Glaser BM, Thompson JT, Sjaarda RN, Pappas SS, Murphy RP. Vitrectomy, fluid-gas exchange and transforming growth factor–beta-2 for the treatment of traumatic macular holes. Ophthalmology. 1995;102(12):1840–5.
73. Garcia-Arumi J, Corcostegui B, Cavero L, Sararols L. The role of vitreoretinal surgery in the treatment of posttraumatic macular hole. Retina (Philadelphia, PA). 1997;17(5):372–7.
74. Colyer MH, Weber ED, Weichel ED, et al. Delayed intraocular foreign body removal without endophthalmitis during Operations Iraqi Freedom and Enduring Freedom. Ophthalmology. 2007;114(8):1439–47.
75. Boldt HC, Pulido JS, Blodi CF, Folk JC, Weingeist TA. Rural endophthalmitis. Ophthalmology. 1989;96(12):1722–6.
76. Narang S, Gupta V, Simalandhi P, Gupta A, Raj S, Dogra MR. Paediatric open globe injuries. Visual outcome and risk factors for endophthalmitis. Indian J Ophthalmol. 2004;52(1):29–34.
77. Alfaro DV, Roth DB, Laughlin RM, Goyal M, Liggett PE. Paediatric post-traumatic endophthalmitis. Br J Ophthalmol. 1995;79(10):888–91.
78. Bhagat N, Nagori S, Zarbin M. Post-traumatic infectious endophthalmitis. Surv Ophthalmol. 2011;56(3):214–51.
79. Essex RW, Yi Q, Charles PG, Allen PJ. Post-traumatic endophthalmitis. Ophthalmology. 2004;111(11):2015–22.
80. Thompson JT, Parver LM, Enger CL, Mieler WF, Liggett PE. Infectious endophthalmitis after penetrating injuries with retained intraocular foreign bodies. National Eye Trauma System. Ophthalmology. 1993;100(10):1468–74.
81. Farr AK, Hairston RJ, Humayun MU, et al. Open globe injuries in children: a retrospective analysis. J Pediatr Ophthalmol Strabismus. 2001;38(2):72–7.
82. Thordsen JE, Harris L, Hubbard 3rd GB. Pediatric endophthalmitis. A 10-year consecutive series. Retina (Philadelphia, PA). 2008;28(3 Suppl):S3–7.

83. Results of the Endophthalmitis Vitrectomy Study. A randomized trial of immediate vitrectomy and of intravenous antibiotics for the treatment of postoperative bacterial endophthalmitis. Endophthalmitis Vitrectomy Study Group. Arch Ophthalmol (Chicago, IL: 1960). 1995;113(12):1479–96.
84. Shah MA, Shah SM, Applewar A, Patel C, Patel K. Ocular Trauma Score as a predictor of final visual outcomes in traumatic cataract cases in pediatric patients. J Cataract Refract Surg. 2012;38(6):959–65.
85. Khokhar S, Gupta S, Yogi R, Gogia V, Agarwal T. Epidemiology and intermediate-term outcomes of open- and closed-globe injuries in traumatic childhood cataract. Eur J Ophthalmol. 2014;24(1):124–30.
86. Reddy AK, Ray R, Yen KG. Surgical intervention for traumatic cataracts in children: epidemiology, complications, and outcomes. J AAPOS (The Official Publication of the American Association for Pediatric Ophthalmology and Strabismus/American Association for Pediatric Ophthalmology and Strabismus). 2009;13(2):170–4.
87. Churchill AJ, Noble BA, Etchells DE, George NJ. Factors affecting visual outcome in children following uniocular traumatic cataract. Eye (London, England). 1995;9(Pt 3):285–91.
88. Binkhorst CD, Gobin MH. Treatment of congenital and juvenile cataract with intraocular lens implants (pseudophakoi). Br J Ophthalmol. 1970;54(11):759–65.
89. Gupta AK, Grover AK, Gurha N. Traumatic cataract surgery with intraocular lens implantation in children. J Pediatr Ophthalmol Strabismus. 1992;29(2):73–8.
90. Gradin D, Yorston D. Intraocular lens implantation for traumatic cataract in children in East Africa. J Cataract Refract Surg. 2001;27(12):2017–25.
91. Zwaan J, Mullaney PB, Awad A, al-Mesfer S, Wheeler DT. Pediatric intraocular lens implantation. Surgical results and complications in more than 300 patients. Ophthalmology. 1998;105(1):112–8; discussion 8–9.
92. BenEzra D, Cohen E, Rose L. Traumatic cataract in children: correction of aphakia by contact lens or intraocular lens. Am J Ophthalmol. 1997;123(6):773–82.
93. Kuchle M, Lausen B, Gusek-Schneider GC. Results and complications of hydrophobic acrylic vs PMMA posterior chamber lenses in children under 17 years of age. Graefes Arch Clin Exp Ophthalmol (Albrecht von Graefes Archiv fur klinische und experimentelle Ophthalmologie). 2003;241(8):637–41.
94. Kugelberg M, Kugelberg U, Bobrova N, Tronina S, Zetterstrom C. After-cataract in children having cataract surgery with or without anterior vitrectomy implanted with a single-piece AcrySof IOL. J Cataract Refract Surg. 2005;31(4):757–62.
95. Sminia ML, Odenthal MT, Wenniger-Prick LJ, Gortzak-Moorstein N, Volker-Dieben HJ. Traumatic pediatric cataract: a decade of follow-up after Artisan aphakia intraocular lens implantation. J AAPOS (The Official Publication of the American Association for Pediatric Ophthalmology and Strabismus/American Association for Pediatric Ophthalmology and Strabismus). 2007;11(6):555–8.
96. Bardorf CM, Epley KD, Lueder GT, Tychsen L. Pediatric transscleral sutured intraocular lenses: efficacy and safety in 43 eyes followed an average of 3 years. J AAPOS. 2004;8:318–24.
97. Buckley EG. Safety of transscleral-sutured intraocular lenses in children. J AAPOS. 2008;12(5):431–9.
98. Enyedi LB, Peterseim MW, Freedman SF, Buckley EG. Refractive changes after pediatric intraocular lens implantation. Am J Ophthalmol. 1998;126(6):772–81.
99. Plager DA, Kipfer H, Sprunger DT, Sondhi N, Neely DE. Refractive change in pediatric pseudophakia: 6-year follow-up. J Cataract Refract Surg. 2002;28(5):810–5.
100. Awner S, Buckley EG, DeVaro JM, Seaber JH. Unilateral pseudophakia in children under 4 years. J Pediatr Ophthalmol Strabismus. 1996;33(4):230–6.
101. Nihalani BR, Vanderveen DK. Secondary intraocular lens implantation after pediatric aphakia. J AAPOS (The Official Publication of the American Association for Pediatric Ophthalmology and Strabismus/American Association for Pediatric Ophthalmology and Strabismus). 2011;15(5):435–40.
102. Solebo AL, Russell-Eggitt I, Cumberland PM, Rahi JS. Risks and outcomes associated with primary intraocular lens implantation in children under 2 years of age: the IoLunder2 cohort study. Br J Ophthalmol. 2015;99(11):1471–6.
103. Lundvall A, Zetterstrom C. Primary intraocular lens implantation in infants: complications and visual results. J Cataract Refract Surg. 2006;32(10):1672–7.
104. Carrigan AK, DuBois LG, Becker ER, Lambert SR. Cost of intraocular lens versus contact lens treatment after unilateral congenital cataract surgery: retrospective analysis at age 1 year. Ophthalmology. 2013;120(1):14–9.
105. Plager DA, Lynn MJ, Buckley EG, Wilson ME, Lambert SR. Complications in the first 5 years following cataract surgery in infants with and without intraocular lens implantation in the Infant Aphakia Treatment Study. Am J Ophthalmol. 2014;158(5):892–8.
106. Gordon RA, Donzis PB. Refractive development of the human eye. Arch Ophthalmol (Chicago, IL: 1960). 1985;103(6):785–9.
107. McClatchey SK, Parks MM. Myopic shift after cataract removal in childhood. J Pediatr Ophthalmol Strabismus. 1997;34(2):88–95.
108. Sorkin JA, Lambert SR. Longitudinal changes in axial length in pseudophakic children. J Cataract Refract Surg. 1997;23 Suppl 1:624–8.
109. Griener ED, Dahan E, Lambert SR. Effect of age at time of cataract surgery on subsequent axial length growth in infant eyes. J Cataract Refract Surg. 1999;25(9):1209–13.

110. O'Keefe M, Fenton S, Lanigan B. Visual outcomes and complications of posterior chamber intraocular lens implantation in the first year of life. J Cataract Refract Surg. 2001;27(12):2006–11.
111. Dahan E, Drusedau MU. Choice of lens and dioptric power in pediatric pseudophakia. J Cataract Refract Surg. 1997;23 Suppl 1:618–23.
112. Crouch ER, Crouch Jr ER, Pressman SH. Prospective analysis of pediatric pseudophakia: myopic shift and postoperative outcomes. J AAPOS (The Official Publication of the American Association for Pediatric Ophthalmology and Strabismus/American Association for Pediatric Ophthalmology and Strabismus). 2002;6(5):277–82.
113. McClatchey SK, Parks MM. Theoretic refractive changes after lens implantation in childhood. Ophthalmology. 1997;104(11):1744–51.
114. Superstein R, Archer SM, Del Monte MA. Minimal myopic shift in pseudophakic versus aphakic pediatric cataract patients. J AAPOS (The Official Publication of the American Association for Pediatric Ophthalmology and Strabismus/American Association for Pediatric Ophthalmology and Strabismus). 2002;6(5):271–6.
115. Tartarella MB, Carani JC, Scarpi MJ. The change in axial length in the pseudophakic eye compared to the unoperated fellow eye in children with bilateral cataracts. J AAPOS (The Official Publication of the American Association for Pediatric Ophthalmology and Strabismus/American Association for Pediatric Ophthalmology and Strabismus). 2014;18(2):173–7.
116. Ahmadieh H, Javadi MA. Intra-ocular lens implantation in children. Curr Opin Ophthalmol. 2001;12(1):30–4.
117. Stager Jr DR, Wang X, Weakley Jr DR, Felius J. The effectiveness of Nd: YAG laser capsulotomy for the treatment of posterior capsule opacification in children with acrylic intraocular lenses. J AAPOS (The Official Publication of the American Association for Pediatric Ophthalmology and Strabismus/American Association for Pediatric Ophthalmology and Strabismus). 2006;10(2):159–63.
118. Hutcheson KA, Drack AV, Ellish NJ, Lambert SR. Anterior hyaloid face opacification after pediatric Nd: YAG laser capsulotomy. J AAPOS (The Official Publication of the American Association for Pediatric Ophthalmology and Strabismus/American Association for Pediatric Ophthalmology and Strabismus). 1999;3(5):303–7.
119. Gimbel HV, DeBroff BM. Posterior capsulorhexis with optic capture: maintaining a clear visual axis after pediatric cataract surgery. J Cataract Refract Surg. 1994;20(6):658–64.
120. Koch DD, Kohnen T. Retrospective comparison of techniques to prevent secondary cataract formation after posterior chamber intraocular lens implantation in infants and children. J Cataract Refract Surg. 1997;23 Suppl 1:657–63.
121. Pandey SK, Wilson ME, Trivedi RH, et al. Pediatric cataract surgery and intraocular lens implantation: current techniques, complications, and management. Int Ophthalmol Clin. 2001;41(3):175–96.
122. Vasavada A, Desai J. Primary posterior capsulorhexis with and without anterior vitrectomy in congenital cataracts. J Cataract Refract Surg. 1997;23 Suppl 1:645–51.
123. Verma N, Ram J, Sukhija J, Pandav SS, Gupta A. Outcome of in-the-bag implanted square-edge polymethyl methacrylate intraocular lenses with and without primary posterior capsulotomy in pediatric traumatic cataract. Indian J Ophthalmol. 2011;59(5):347–51.
124. Agrawal R, Shah M, Mireskandari K, Yong GK. Controversies in ocular trauma classification and management: review. Int Ophthalmol. 2013;33(4):435–45.
125. Hsu HT, Ryan SJ. Natural history of penetrating ocular injury with retinal laceration in the monkey. Graefes Arch Clin Exp Ophthalmol (Albrecht von Graefes Archiv fur klinische und experimentelle Ophthalmologie). 1986;224(1):1–6.
126. Cleary PE, Ryan SJ. Method of production and natural history of experimental posterior penetrating eye injury in the rhesus monkey. Am J Ophthalmol. 1979;88(2):212–20.
127. Sandinha MT, Newman W, Wong D, Stappler T. Outcomes of delayed vitrectomy in open-globe injuries in young patients. Retina (Philadelphia, PA). 2011;31(8):1541–4.
128. Hermsen V. Vitrectomy in severe ocular trauma. Ophthalmologica (Journal International d'ophtalmologie International Journal of Ophthalmology Zeitschrift fur Augenheilkunde). 1984;189(1–2):86–92.
129. Vatne HO, Syrdalen P. Vitrectomy in double perforating eye injuries. Acta Ophthalmol (Copenh). 1985;63(5):552–6.
130. Ahmadieh H, Soheilian M, Sajjadi H, Azarmina M, Abrishami M. Vitrectomy in ocular trauma. Factors influencing final visual outcome. Retina (Philadelphia, PA). 1993;13(2):107–13.
131. Dalma-Weiszhausz J, Quiroz-Mercado H, Morales-Canton V, Oliver-Fernandez K, De Anda-Turati M. Vitrectomy for ocular trauma: a question of timing? Eur J Ophthalmol. 1996;6(4):460–3.
132. Wong SC, Capone Jr A. Microplasmin (ocriplasmin) in pediatric vitreoretinal surgery: update and review. Retina (Philadelphia, PA). 2013;33(2):339–48.

7 Severe Traumatic Eyes with No Light Perception

Haoyu Chen, Honghe Xia, and Danny Siu-Chun Ng

7.1 Introduction

Severe open globe ocular injury may result in no light perception (NLP) at presentation. It is important to confirm the visual acuity of NLP. The assessment of light perception should be performed in a dark room, the contralateral eye should be covered completely, the light of the indirect ophthalmoscopy should be turned to maximal intensity, and the distance from the indirect ophthalmoscopy to the eye should be kept sufficient to prevent that the patient perceives the heat of the light.

It is well established that NLP at presentation suggests poor outcome. The Ocular Trauma Score (OTS) was validated using data from over 2500 cases from national eye injury registries to predict outcome of ocular trauma, in which NLP and afferent pupillary defect (APD) had the poorest outcome; 74 % of patients with NLP after open globe injury were irreversible [1]. Besides blindness, severe traumatic eyes may subsequently lead to pain due to phthisis bulbi. Furthermore, there is risk of sympathetic ophthalmia in the contralateral eye, potentially leading to vision loss in the uninjured eye because of inflammation, glaucoma, cataract, and retinal detachment.

As a result, severe traumatic eyes may require enucleation or evisceration. However, controversies exist over the management of these severe traumatic eyes with NLP because some of this kind of eye can be saved and even recover some vision. In this chapter, we will discuss the current issues on the management of severe traumatic eyes with NLP.

H. Chen, MD, PhD (✉) • H. Xia
Joint Shantou International Eye Center, Shantou University and the Chinese University of Hong Kong, Shantou, China
e-mail: drchenhaoyu@gmail.com

D.S.-C. Ng
Department of Ophthalmology and Visual Sciences, The Chinese University of Hong Kong, Hong Kong, China

7.2 Current Consensuses on Traumatic Blind Eyes

Most ophthalmologists agree that the primary management of traumatic eye with open globe with NLP should be tried to repair rather than enucleation or evisceration [2]. The reasons are listed as follows:

1. The assessment of NLP is a subjective measure and may be affected by psychological status. Patients may suffer from severe pain and cannot cooperate with visual acuity examination. Some patients may be unconscious, under the influence of mind-altering substances, which made the assessment impossible or unreliable. Some patients may be hysterical or were malingering, and the result of assessment is misleading.

H. Yan (ed.), *Mechanical Ocular Trauma*, DOI 10.1007/978-981-10-2150-3_7

2. Loss of light perception may be caused by many factors, including severe optic media opacity, optic nerve injury by optic canal fracture, massive chorioretinal or suprachoroidal hemorrhage, ophthalmic artery occlusion or central retinal artery occlusion, and extensive retinal and/or choroidal loss. Severe vitreous hemorrhage can block the light getting into the retina, even with the bright light of indirect ophthalmoscopy [3, 4]. Although APD, electroretinography, and visual evoked potential are objective assessment of the damage of the retina and optic nerve, the results may also be false positive in the presence of severe hyphema or vitreous hemorrhage [5, 6]. Medial opacity can be amenable by surgical intervention to recover some visual function.
3. The loss of light perception after open globe injury may be transient. Salehi-Had [7] reported that in 88 cases with open globe injury and the presenting vision was NLP, 23 (26.1 %) spontaneously recover to at least light perception after primary repair. With advances of vitreoretinal surgery, a significant proportion of cases can be salvaged. We will discuss this point later.
4. Patients may have impaired consciousness, caused by trauma of the brain, psychological stress, or affected by mind-altering substances. This may affect the obtaining of informed consent of primary enucleation or evisceration. Primary repair of the wound allows time for the recovery of consciousness and obtaining of informed consent for secondary enucleation or further intraocular surgery. According to a telephone survey, most of the patients who had suffered from open globe injuries would not want to consider primary enucleation, even if it could avoid further surgery [8]. When possible, allow some time for the patient to realize and accept that his or her eye is no longer functional.
5. It was found that the incidence of sympathetic ophthalmia is low. The reported incidence after open globe injury is 0–0.9 % in recent literature [9, 10]. Furthermore, even if sympathetic ophthalmia develops, corticosteroid or immunosuppressive agents can control the inflammation and save the vision. Therefore, prevention of sympathetic ophthalmia should not be a reason for primary enucleation or evisceration.

7.3 Current Controversies and Alternative Management on Severe Traumatic Eyes with NLP

Primary repair is generally accepted, however, subsequent management of these eyes after primary repair remains controversial. The options include enucleation/evisceration, observation, and vitreoretinal surgery.

Conventionally, it is recommended that the severe open globe-injured eyes be enucleated or eviscerated within 2 weeks to prevent sympathetic ophthalmia [11–13]. However, it is argued that the incidence is very low. Albert and Diaz-Rohena reviewed the historical literature on the penetrating wounds of the eye and noted that the incidence of sympathetic ophthalmia ranged from 0 to 12 % among five series published in the nineteenth century, 0.5 to 3 % in the first half of the twentieth century, and 0.28 to 1.9 % in the second half of the twentieth century [13]. A summary of recently published articles is provided in Table 7.1. The incidence of sympathetic ophthal-

Table 7.1 Recent literatures on incidence of sympathetic ophthalmia after open globe injuries

Article	Years of study	N of injured eyes	N of sympathetic ophthalmia
Rofail 2006 [14]	1992–2003	273	1 (0.4 %)
Casson 2002 [9]	1994–1998	109	1 (0.9 %)
Savar 2009 [15]	2000–2007	660	2 (0.3 %)
du Toit 2008 [16]	1995–2004	1392	2 (0.14 %)
Gürdal 2002 [10]	1970–2000	217	0 (0 %)
Zhang 2009 [17]	2001–2005	9103	18 (0.37 %)
Mansouri 2009 [18]	1998–2003	2340	2 (0.08 %)

Table 7.2 Summary of literature reports on visual outcome of vitreoretinal surgery for open globe ocular injuries with no light perception

Articles	*n*	>=LP	LP	HM	CF-20/400	>=20/400
Hui 1996 [23]	10	6 (60 %)	NR	NR	NR	NR
Dong 2002 [24]	11	7 (63.6 %)	1 (9 %)	3 (27 %)	2 (18 %)	1 (9 %)
Yan 2006 [25]	7	5 (71.4 %)	1 (14.3 %)	2 (28.6 %)	1 (14.3 %)	1 (14.3 %)
Wang 2007 [26]	38	21 (55.3 %)	10 (26.3 %)	3 (7.9 %)	5 (13.2 %)	3 (7.9 %)
Heidari 2010 [22]	18	16 (88.9 %)	3 (16.7 %)	4 (22.2 %)	3 (16.7 %)	6 (33.3 %)
Feng 2011 [27]	33	18 (54.50 %)	4 (12.1 %)	1 (3 %)	8 (24.2 %)	5 (15.2 %)
Agrawal 2012 [28]	27	9 (33.30 %)	NR	NR	NR	NR
Soni 2013 [29]	73	17 (23 %)	5 (6.8 %)	9 (12.3 %)	2 (2.7 %)	1 (1.4 %)
Yang 2013 [30]	19	12 (63.2 %)	3 (15.8 %)	1 (5.3 %)	6 (31.6 %)	2 (10.5 %)
Han 2015 [31]	5	4 (80 %)	1 (20 %)	3 (60 %)	0	0

NR not reported, *LP* light perception, *HM* hand movement, *CF* counting fingers

mia ranged from 0 to 0.9 % in the recent two decades, which is much lower compared to previous results. The reduction of incidence of sympathetic ophthalmia may be due to the advances of microsurgical instruments and techniques in open globe repair. Based on the recent reports, prophylactic enucleations are needed to be performed on at least 100 eyes to prevent a case of sympathetic ophthalmia.

Even when sympathetic ophthalmia develops, most patients can still retain good vision with proper treatment, including corticosteroid and immunomodulators [19]. Castiblanco summarized 86 cases reported in literature and found that 70 % patients had improved visual acuity in the sympathizing eye. Even in 58.2 % patients had a visual acuity of at least 20/40 [20]. Galor reported that within 85 cases with sympathetic ophthalmia, the vision outcome was better than 20/50 in 59 % of the sympathizing eyes and better than 20/200 in 75 % of the sympathizing eyes [19]. Therefore, prophylactic enucleations to prevent sympathetic ophthalmia may not be indicated. It has been reported that time trends in enucleating eyes showed the number of enucleations for trauma had dropped during the 10-year period 1986–1995 compared to 1976–1985 [21].

The second option is observation. Salehi-Had reported that in 88 cases with open globe injury with NLP, 23 (26.1 %) spontaneously recovered to light perception (LP) after primary repair. Among them, eight received vitreoretinal surgery. Finally, five of them gained vision, two remained LP, and the other one was NLP. All the other 15 eyes that did not receive vitrectomy lost light perception or became phthisical [7].

In situations in which the eyes become phthisical and there is persistent pain in the eye, enucleation or evisceration seems inevitable. However, before making a final decision, possible options should be discussed with the patient. Some patients may want to keep their useless eye rather than enucleation or evisceration because the latter option would cause great psychological impact on the patient.

The third option is vitreoretinal surgery. The cause of NLP after open globe injury may be reversible and can be restored by vitreoretinal surgery, such as dense vitreous hemorrhage, retinal detachment, subretinal hemorrhage, etc. With the advances in equipment and techniques in vitreoretinal surgery, these conditions can be successfully managed. It has been reported that some eyes with NLP after severe open globe injury may recover to at least light perception after vitreoretinal surgery. Table 7.2 summarized the literature revealing that 23–88.9 % of patients regained light perception after vitreoretinal surgery. Up to 33.4 % of the patients could even gain vision equal or better than 20/200 [22]. Figures 7.1 and 7.2 demonstrate two cases which

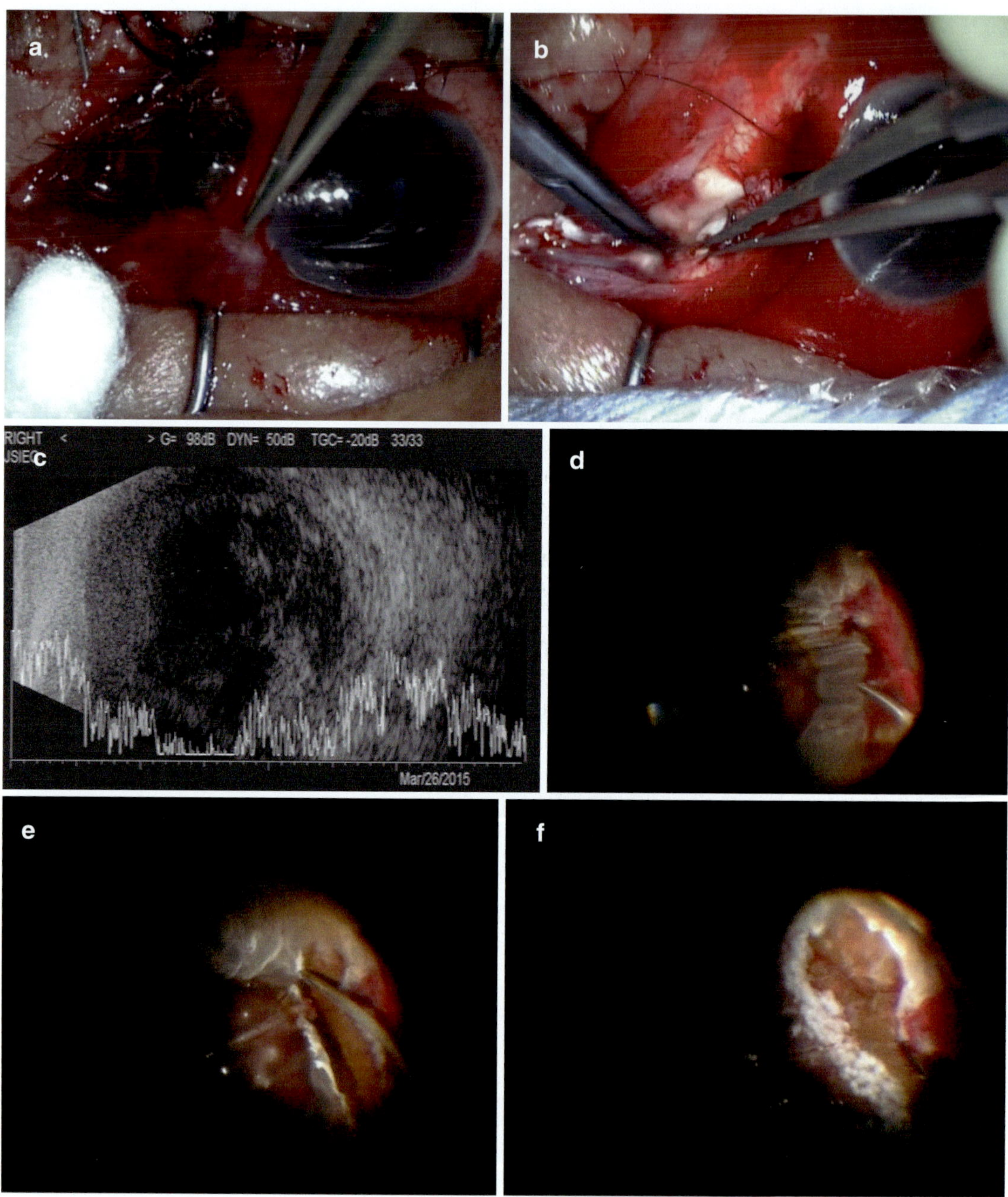

Fig. 7.1 A case recovered from no light perception (NLP) after surgery for open globe injury. A 59-year-old male presented with NLP after assaulted by fist. A scleral rupture was identified 15 mm posterior to the limbus with measured length of 20 mm (**a**, **b**). The wound was repaired immediately. Ultrasound showed signs indicating intraocular hemorrhage, retinal detachment, and choroidal detachment (**c**). Four weeks later, vitreoretinal surgery was performed. After clear of vitreous hemorrhage, retinal incarceration was found at temporal side (**d**). Retinotomy (**e**) and laser photocoagulation (**f**) were performed followed by silicone oil tamponade. The retina was reattached successfully (**g**). Six months later, retina remained attached but an epiretinal membrane developed (**h**, **j**). Five months after silicone oil removal and epiretinal membrane peeling, the retina remained attached (**i**, **k**), and the best corrected visual acuity was 20/160

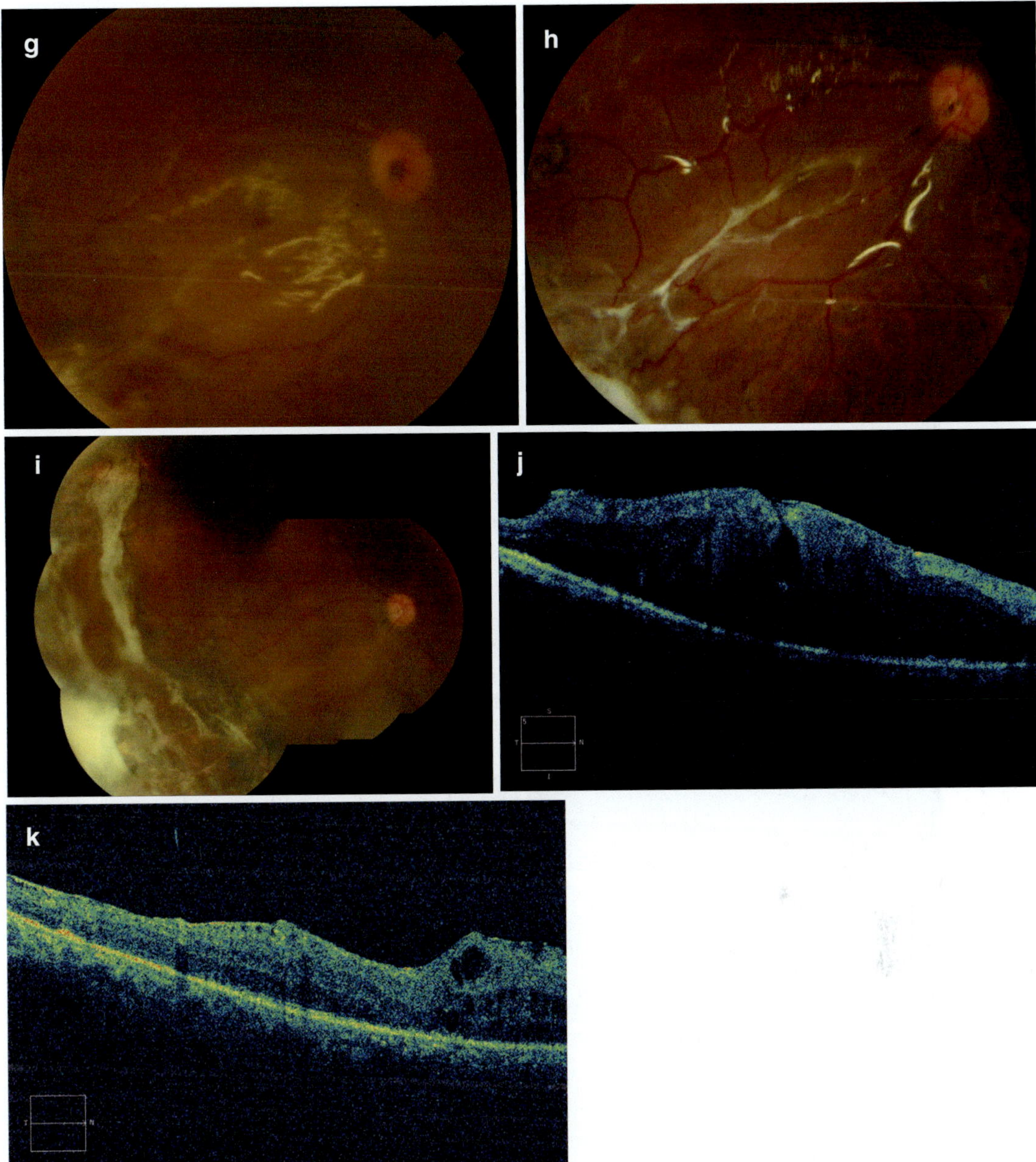

Fig. 7.1 (continued)

recovered from NLP after vitreoretinal surgery for open globe injury.

The surgical procedure may be very complex and challenging. It may include combination of vitrectomy, phacoemulsification or lensectomy, laser photocoagulation, 360° retinotomy, drainage of subretinal hemorrhage and/or suprachoroidal hemorrhage, etc. The surgical field may become blurred by an opaque cornea. Intraocular hemorrhage is difficult to control even with diathermy because the bleeding spot cannot be identified. If the retinal detachment fails to be

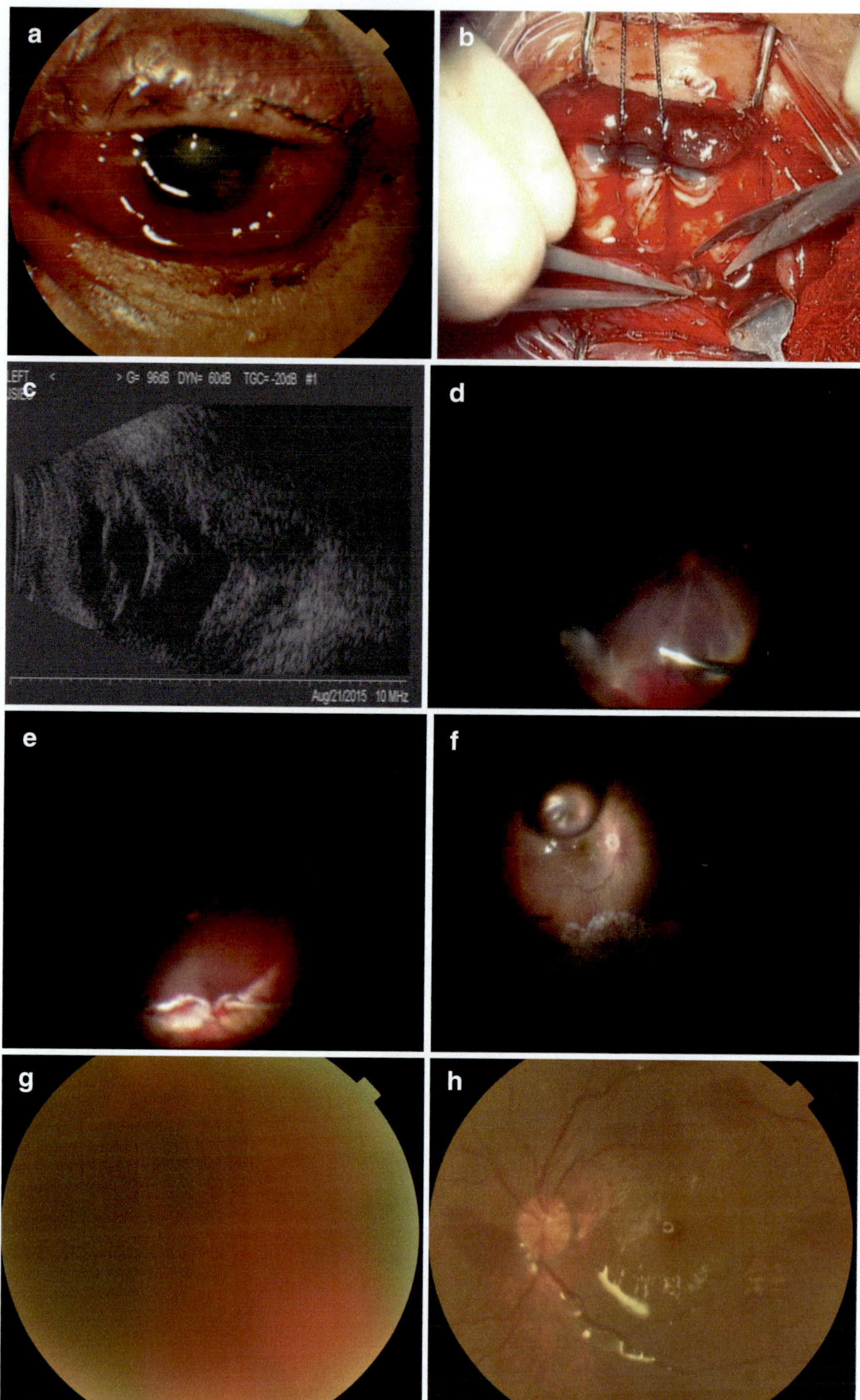

Fig. 7.2 A case recovered from no light perception (NLP) after surgery for open globe injury. A 73-year-old male presented with NLP after assaulted by a fist (**a**). A scleral rupture was 8 mm posterior to the limbus with measured length of 11 mm (**b**). The wound was repaired immediately. There was severe vitreous hemorrhage obscuring fundal view (**g**). Ultrasound showed signs indicating intraocular hemorrhage, retinal detachment, and choroidal detachment (**c**). Eighteen days later, vitreoretinal surgery was performed. After vitrectomy, a retinal incarceration was found superiorly (**d**). Retinotomy (**e**) and laser photocoagulation (**f**) were performed followed by silicone oil tamponade. The retina was flattened (**h**). Six months later, the retina remained attached and the best corrected visual acuity was 20/120

Clinical Pearls for Treatment

1. In primary management, globe-salvaging procedures should always be tried to repair the open globe injury even with NLP. Primary enucleation/evisceration is not recommended.
2. After primary repair, the options of severe traumatic eyes with NLP include enucleation, observation, and vitreoretinal surgery. Assessment of the structure and severity of injury are important for choice management strategy. If the cause of NLP can be repaired by operation, vitreoretinal surgery is indicated. Otherwise, vitrectomy may accelerate phthisis bulbi. Discussion of the advantage and risk of these options with the patients are also important.
3. Secondary enucleation/evisceration is indicated for phthisis bulbi or persistent pain. It is not indicated for prevention of sympathetic ophthalmia because the incidence is extremely low (less than 1 %).
4. Vitreoretinal surgery can restore at least light perception in 23–88.9 % patient with NLP after open globe injury.

flattened, the loss of vitreous support may hasten the development of phthisis bulbi. Therefore, silicone oil tamponade is strongly recommended. Preoperative assessment is very important. And the doctors should also assess his surgical experience. Sometimes, referring the patients to an experienced surgeon might benefit the patient.

The timing of vitreoretinal surgery is also controversial. The advantage of early vitrectomy is to avoid proliferative reaction in the vitreous and retina. However, there may be tight vitreous-retinal adhesion, and it is difficult to induce posterior vitreous detachment during operation. In addition, there may be corneal edema hindering the view during vitreous surgery. Active intraocular hemorrhage during operation can add to the difficulty of surgery. Delayed surgery may help avoid these disadvantages; however, severe proliferative vitreoretinopathy may develop, which may lead to closed funnel retinal detachment. The optimal timing for vitreoretinal surgery in open globe injury is 10 days to 3 weeks. The exception is when there is endophthalmitis or intraocular foreign body with risk of infection, which requires early intervention.

References

1. Kuhn F, et al. The Ocular Trauma Score (OTS). Ophthalmol Clin North Am. 2002;15(2):163–5, vi.
2. Agrawal R, et al. Controversies in ocular trauma classification and management: review. Int Ophthalmol. 2013;33(4):435–45.
3. Morris R, Kuhn F, and Witherspoon CD. Management of the opaque media eye with no light perception. In: Alfaro III DV, Liggett PE, editors. Vitreoretinal surgery of the injured eye. Lippincott Raven: Philadelphia; 1999. p. 113–24.
4. Abrams GW, Knighton RW. Falsely extinguished bright-flash electroretinogram. Its association with dense vitreous hemorrhage. Arch Ophthalmol. 1982;100(9):1427–9.
5. Striph GG, et al. Afferent pupillary defect caused by hyphema. Am J Ophthalmol. 1988;106(3):352–3.
6. Mandelbaum S, et al. Bright-flash electroretinography and vitreous hemorrhage. An experimental study in primates. Arch Ophthalmol. 1980;98(10):1823–8.
7. Salehi-Had H, et al. Visual outcomes of vitreoretinal surgery in eyes with severe open-globe injury presenting with no-light-perception vision. Graefes Arch Clin Exp Ophthalmol. 2009;247(4):477–83.
8. Rofail M, Lee GA, O'Rourke P. Quality of life after open-globe injury. Ophthalmology. 2006;113(6):1057.e1–3.
9. Casson RJ, Walker JC, Newland HS. Four-year review of open eye injuries at the Royal Adelaide Hospital. Clin Experiment Ophthalmol. 2002;30(1):15–8.
10. Gurdal C, et al. Incidence of sympathetic ophthalmia after penetrating eye injury and choice of treatment. Ocul Immunol Inflamm. 2002;10(3):223–7.
11. Chan CK, Chhablani J, Freeman WR. Prognostic indicators for no light perception after open-globe injury: eye injury vitrectomy study. Am J Ophthalmol. 2012;153(4):777, author reply 778.
12. Chu DS, Foster CS. Sympathetic ophthalmia. Int Ophthalmol Clin. 2002;42(3):179–85.
13. Albert DM, Diaz-Rohena R. A historical review of sympathetic ophthalmia and its epidemiology. Surv Ophthalmol. 1989;34(1):1–14.
14. Rofail M, Lee GA, O'Rourke P. Prognostic indicators for open globe injury. Clin Experiment Ophthalmol. 2006;34(8):783–6.
15. Savar A, et al. Enucleation for open globe injury. Am J Ophthalmol. 2009;147(4):595–600.e1.
16. du Toit N, et al. The risk of sympathetic ophthalmia following evisceration for penetrating eye injuries at

Groote Schuur Hospital. Br J Ophthalmol. 2008;92(1): 61–3.
17. Zhang Y, et al. Development of sympathetic ophthalmia following globe injury. Chin Med J (Engl). 2009;122(24):2961–6.
18. Mansouri M, et al. Epidemiology of open-globe injuries in Iran: analysis of 2,340 cases in 5 years (report no. 1). Retina. 2009;29(8):1141–9.
19. Galor A, et al. Sympathetic ophthalmia: incidence of ocular complications and vision loss in the sympathizing eye. Am J Ophthalmol. 2009;148(5):704–10.e2.
20. Castiblanco CP, Adelman RA. Sympathetic ophthalmia. Graefes Arch Clin Exp Ophthalmol. 2009;247(3):289–302.
21. Gunalp I, Gunduz K, Ozkan M. Causes of enucleation: a clinicopathological study. Eur J Ophthalmol. 1997;7(3):223–8.
22. Heidari E, Taheri N. Surgical treatment of severely traumatized eyes with no light perception. Retina. 2010;30(2):294–9.
23. Hui Y, Wang L, Shan W. Exploratory vitrectomy for traumatized eyes with no light perception and dense vitreous hemorrhage. Zhonghua Yan Ke Za Zhi. 1996;32(6):450–2.
24. Dong F, Dai R. The surgical treatment of traumatized eyes with no light perception. Zhonghua Yan Ke Za Zhi. 2002;38(11):657–9.
25. Yan H, et al. Penetrating keratoplasty combined with vitreoretinal surgery for severe ocular injury with blood-stained cornea and no light perception. Ophthalmologica. 2006;220(3):186–9.
26. Wang YN, et al. Prognosis of traumatic eyes with no light perception undergone vitrectomy and analysis of risk factors. Zhonghua Yan Ke Za Zhi. 2007;43(4):340–5.
27. Feng K, Hu YT, Ma Z. Prognostic indicators for no light perception after open-globe injury: eye injury vitrectomy study. Am J Ophthalmol. 2011;152(4):654–62. e2.
28. Agrawal R, Wei HS, Teoh S. Predictive factors for final outcome of severely traumatized eyes with no light perception. BMC Ophthalmol. 2012;12:16.
29. Soni NG, et al. Open globe ocular trauma: functional outcome of eyes with no light perception at initial presentation. Retina. 2013;33(2):380–6.
30. Yang SS, Jiang T. Vitrectomy combined with silicone oil tamponade in the treatment of severely traumatized eyes with the visual acuity of no light perception. Int J Ophthalmol. 2013;6(2):198–203.
31. Han YS, Kavoussi SC, Adelman RA. Visual recovery following open globe injury with initial no light perception. Clin Ophthalmol. 2015;9:1443–8.

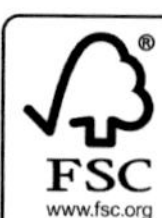

MIX
Papier aus verantwortungsvollen Quellen
Paper from responsible sources
FSC® C105338

If you have any concerns about our products, you can contact us on
ProductSafety@springernature.com

In case Publisher is established outside the EU, the EU authorized representative is:
Springer Nature Customer Service Center GmbH
Europaplatz 3, 69115 Heidelberg, Germany

Printed by Libri Plureos GmbH
in Hamburg, Germany